Close Encounters
of the Bovine

Close Encounters
of the Bovine

Recollections of a Rural Veterinarian

Rosalie Cooper-Chase, DVM
Foreword by Mark Rashid

Johnson Books, Boulder
Spring Creek Press, Estes Park

Published by Johnson Books, a division of Big Earth Publishing, 3005 Center Green Drive, Suite 220, Boulder, Colorado 80301. www.johnsonbooks.com

Composition by D. Kari Luraas, Clairvoyance Design.
Cover design by Polly Christensen.
Cover photo by Jack Chase. The bovine belongs to the Rocking L Ranch, Kennard, TX.

9 8 7 6 5 4 3 2 1

Library of Congress Cataloging-in-Publication Data
Cooper-Chase, Rosalie.
    Close encounters of the bovine: recollections of a rural veterinarian/Rosalie Cooper-Chase.
        p. cm.
    ISBN 1-55566-378-8
1. Cooper-Chase, Rosalie. 2. Veterinarians—Texas—Biography. 3. Women veterinarians—Texas—Biography. 4. Veterinary medicine—Texas—Anecdotes. 5. Cattle—Diseases—Texas—Anecdotes. I. Title.
    SF613.C66C66 2006
    636.089092-dc22

                                                                                        2006004136

Printed in the United States of America

This book is dedicated to
all my friends and family who said to me,
"You should write these things down!"
Thank you for your love and support.
And to my parents, who taught us by example
how to treat all creatures, human and otherwise.
I love you, Dad. I miss you, Mom.

Contents

Foreword
by Mark Rashid

I had just finished reading the manuscript of this book, *Close Encounters of the Bovine*, when I happened to mention it to a friend who has absolutely no background in livestock whatsoever. When I told him I had read this wonderful book about cattle, a truly perplexed look crossed his face.

I must say, his expression spoke volumes. It began with a slight wrinkling of his brow; then came a flaring of his nostrils, like you would do if you had just stepped in something unpleasant. After that, his expression slowly switched to one of bewilderment, as if the words "wonderful book" and "cattle" somehow didn't (nor would they ever) fit together comfortably in the same sentence. I suppose there are more than just a few folks out there who might feel the same way.

To those folks, all I can say is—you're in for a pleasant surprise!

❖

I met Dr. Rosalie Cooper-Chase many years ago when she came to ride one of her horses in a clinic I was conducting in Texas. One of the first things I noticed about her then—and continue to see in her to this day—is her total and unmitigated compassion for animals of all kinds. What I have come to understand over the years, however, is that she holds a particularly soft spot in her heart for those animals she writes about so eloquently in this book … cattle.

You see, Rosalie understands the truth about cattle, a truth known mostly by devoted stockmen and women, along with dedicated veterinarians, like Dr. Rosalie.

❖

There was a time, not really all that long ago, when cattle were king out here in the West and in a few other parts of the country, as well. Back then, before urban sprawl and cell phones and automobiles and paved roads and fences, fortunes (and lives) were made, and sometimes lost, over cattle. Railroads built tracks westward, and towns and cities sprouted up because of cattle. Huge tracts of land were eventually gobbled up by the cattle barons (usually where the best water could be found), and on those tracts grazed vast herds of cattle, many gathered in Texas and brought north to populate the plains that once held buffalo, by then nearly extinct.

The herds of cattle in the West eventually became so big that an easterner traveling through the West in the mid-1880s wrote home saying one could hardly throw a rock on the prairie without hitting a bovine of some kind.

Unfortunately (or fortunately depending on what side of the fence one stands on), those days are long gone. And, while there are cattle operations still going strong in many places around the country, I believe it's safe to say the true heyday of the cattle business is pretty much over. One of the most regrettable things about this is that along with the disappearance of many of the country's large and small ranches and cattle operations also goes the loss of many of the men and women who carried with them the knowledge and understanding of the cattle they tended.

What Rosalie has so aptly done in this book is given us a glimpse of a time and a way of life that may someday be gone from our landscape. It's a snapshot of people, places, and animals that, sadly, are quickly disappearing from our consciousness. The stories in this book are bound to have a profound effect on those who read them, regardless of whether you've spent countless miles in the saddle staring at the south end of northbound cattle or you've only encountered cows when you've seen them standing in a pasture as you drive by at sixty-five miles per hour.

❖

Undoubtedly, some of the stories you are about to read will make you smile. Some of them may cause you to shed a tear; and others may make you feel downright uncomfortable. Still, in the end what shines through all of them is not only Dr. Rosalie's compassion for her charges, her respect for the humans involved, and her ability to treat both with dignity, but also the honor and integrity with which her work was performed.

My guess is by the time you've finished reading *Close Encounters of the Bovine*, you will hope, the same way so many others already do, that if one of your animals were in trouble, someone like Dr. Rosalie Cooper-Chase would already be in a truck heading your way.

❖

Mark Rashid is known for his unique ability to understand and communicate with horses. He presents horsemanship clinics across the country and around the world. He is the author of five books: Considering the Horse: Tales of Problems Solved and Lessons Learned; A Good Horse is Never a Bad Color; Horses Never Lie: The Heart of Passive Leadership; Life Lessons from a Ranch Horse; *and* Horsemanship Through Life. *He still works cattle at a ranch near his home in Estes Park, Colorado.*

Preface

These are stories about some work I did attending cattle in distress. For the first fourteen years or so as a licensed veterinarian, I was a mixed-animal practitioner; that is, I worked with just about any animal that needed help, although mostly it meant dogs and cats, horses and cattle, a few swine, and an occasional goat or sheep. A few years ago, I was forced to give up my large-animal practice due to a couple of serious injuries, although I still keep a few head of cattle and ride my horses.

Horses were why I got into veterinary medicine—horses and cats. I love cats. My love of those two species was the main reason I sweated through years of pre-veterinary medicine courses, why I struggled through veterinary college, why I wanted to be employed only in mixed practices once I got out, and why I have had and still have so many horses and cats.

Ah, but cows. Why a book about cows? Why did I want to work with cows to begin with? I didn't grow up around cattle. Our family didn't have cows; actually, the milk we drank usually came in a powdered form. I didn't know much about cattle in general before I helped milk a couple of dairy cows and fed the milk to a few feeder calves when I was a teenager.

I really learned about cows, grew to like them, appreciate them, and want to work with them, when I was employed as a veterinary assistant in my twenties. Regular people don't get up close and personal with many cows, certainly not like they do with dogs or kittens. Due to this lack of interaction, cows get a bum rap in public relations. Cows are not considered to be very smart. They appear only to stand around a lot, eating grass. Cows are thought to be good for mainly just three things—milk, meat, and leather. However, cows are very good at being what they are; no other animal on earth is as good at being bovine as is a cow. For what they were designed to be, cows are the best.

One of the things that drew me into veterinary medicine was my empathy for animals, all animals. In my veterinary practice it was my desire to do the best thing in each case I was presented with. It was often not an easy job, and not all the owners of the animals I tended cared as much for the animals' comfort and well-being as I thought they should have. I viewed animals not as lesser beings but as creatures no less deserving of compassion and consideration than is the human species.

My own opinion about animals—and it really doesn't matter to me if you agree with me or not—was and is that animals were created, yes, for our use, but firstly to make God happy. And I'm sure that they do just that and do it very well. They go about their business honestly, being the best at what they were created to be.

Animals would seem to have no desires other than to be comfortable and well fed, with the kindness and the friendship of fellow creatures as a bonus. Animals do not aspire to wealth; a cardboard box with an old towel thrown in it is just as satisfying to a purebred Persian cat as it is to a ragged old alley cat. Dogs are perfectly content to hang out with their packs, canine or human, with no regard to whether the house is a mansion in town or a shack in the woods. A horse would rather have the company of his mates in a field open to the extremes of the weather than the loneliness of the most luxurious stall.

And a cow never barters her milk and offspring for feed and a stall. She only asks to be treated fairly and with dignity. And what's wrong with that?

These stories are little slices of my life as a large-animal practitioner in East Texas. Most of my clients who owned cattle had only a few head, and they liked their cows, not only as a source of income but as companion travelers on this planet. I appreciated those clients most who considered their animals first, who didn't really think about how much it might cost before they called on my assistance to restore the cow's health or save a calf. I liked that about those people, as it made my job easier and enjoyable.

To see a newborn calf lying on the ground, struggling for his first breath, to witness his first sight of the wide world and his first attempt to stand and nurse, to know I saved his life and probably his mother's also—that was good stuff. Diagnosing and successfully treating a sick, suffering animal and knowing that I had a hand in its recovery was a totally exhilarating and also humbling experience. I loved my job.

So, to all those people who love their animals, who treat them with dignity and respect, thank you. To all those animals who forgive us our clumsiness in our attempts to help them, thank you. And as we travel this good earth together, may God be happy with us all.

Part 1

Unspoken

Communication

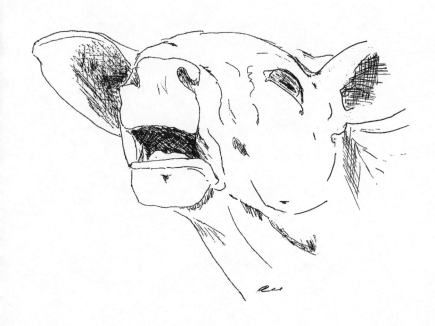

Loading Mr. Martin's Cow

An animal's eyes have the power to speak a great language.
—Martin Buber

I firmly believed that I was able to do my job as well as I did not only because of the excellent training I had in veterinary school and my real-world experience, but also because of my deep respect and empathy for animals. What many people do not realize is that animals have an uncanny ability to read us humans, our body language, and our intentions toward them that we are not even aware we display.

When I worked with cattle and other animals, I tried to do so with a great deal of regard for their discomfort and fear of the situation. Combined with something that I can only describe as spiritual, working with cattle was often an amazing experience for me. Such was the case with Mr. Martin's cow.

Why some cows pick cold, wet days to usher their newborns into the world is a puzzle to me. It does seem that, more often than not, the cows attempting to calve on cold, wet days need assistance. Maybe it's because the cold-weather calves just have less desire to slide out onto frozen ground than the calves born on more temperate days. It could even be that we veterinarians are just a little more reluctant to go out in inclement weather, and

3

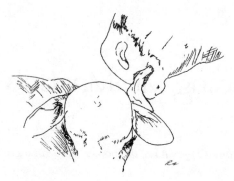

that makes the bad-weather deliveries seem more grueling and numerous. For whatever reasons, the nasty weather calvings seem to be stored in the memory banks with a little more detail than are their fair-weather counterparts.

Mr. Martin had a small herd of cows in a pasture situated about twenty miles from town, and getting to his place entailed traveling some unimproved back roads. So, when he called one cold, blustery morning to ask for assistance with a heifer in dystocia—a ten-dollar word that means "difficult birth"—it was all I could do to suppress a moan. Could he possibly trailer her to the clinic? No, that wasn't possible. His trailer was in the shop having the floorboards replaced. He expected that I'd have to go out to see the cow.

I'll admit, it was with great reluctance that I climbed into my truck for the drive out to the Martins' place. Besides being in the middle of nowhere, the ranch was situated along the river bottom, smack in the middle of some of the lowest-lying land in the county. After a rain, water stayed on that ground forever. We'd recently had some torrential rains, and I figured the ranch would be ankle-deep in water, mud, and mire. To add to the attraction of the place, pens were non-existent. Mr. Martin depended on stout ropes and nearby trees or fence posts to restrain cattle needing work. How he managed to load cattle for a trip to the sale barn was unknown to me.

Now I had a call to go out there and help a struggling cow. I sighed, pulled my coat around me just a little tighter, put the truck in gear, and began my journey to the ranch at the end of the world.

❖

The drive out was as I expected—the road up to the ranch was slick with mud and treacherous. Mr. Martin met me at the gate with his tractor and a tow chain—always a bad sign. He signaled that I should follow. I put the truck in low gear and moved down the lane behind the tractor. We seemed to be surrounded by water, with the only high point being the roadbed over which we slowly traveled. A fine mist of rain was falling, adding to the gloom of the day.

I kept my eyes on the old man where he sat ramrod straight in the metal seat of an ancient tractor that popped and farted exhaust into the chilly air. Mr. Martin raised his hand to indicate a stop, and I allowed the mud sucking on the tires to pull my Dodge to a standstill. Since he was climbing down from the tractor, I guessed I should join him. I opened the door and slid off the seat, dropping my rubber-booted feet into frigid water three inches deep. I slogged over to where Mr. Martin stood at the front of his tractor. On the roadbed about fifty feet ahead lay a cow, miserable in the cold, huge with an unborn calf, her legs stiff and neck arched as she strained to rid herself of the produce of her uterus. I slogged over to check her out.

Nothing showed beneath her tail. I waded back to my truck for OB gloves and lube and then made my way back to the cow. She wore no halter, but a short lariat rope encircled her neck. There was nothing nearby, no tree, no post, to tie it to. However, it was evident that the poor cow was not going to be getting up and running away. She rolled her upside eye to me, the whites showing large. I checked her general condition and cringed at her small size. Mr. Martin had told me the cow was only sixteen months old. She had come into her first heat nine months earlier while still on her own mama, turned out with a big crossbred Hereford bull. She might have weighed 500 pounds without the calf inside her. She was thin and rough-coated, but her udder was strutted, full of milk for the unborn calf. She groaned and strained fruitlessly.

The ground was cold and muddy where I knelt behind the heifer. I shivered as the chill from the ground ran up my knees to the rest of me. I pulled on the shoulder-length plastic OB gloves, cleaned the cow's rear end with soap and the warm water from my gallon jug, lubed up my hands, and inserted my right hand into her vagina, wondering what I would find.

Immediately, my fingers encountered two enormous hoofs encased in the soft, white covering that protects the uterus from injury from the calf's hoofs and, just behind them, the head of a calf, the diameter of which exceeded the diameter of the birth canal. When my fingers tested for a suckle reflex, the calf's response was immediate and strong. Very much alive, but there was no way this calf would enter the world the way God had intended. A Caesarean section was the only way both cow and calf could be saved.

I stood up, stripping off the long OB gloves as I turned to Mr. Martin, who stood silently holding the end of the rope. I must have been tired or cold, or both. For a moment, my mind flashed a picture of the thin old man tethered to this cow who, only in my mind, had leaped up and was galloping frantically across the watery pasture, the rancher still hanging onto the rope, flapping like a pennant in her wake. I shook my head and jumped back into reality. Mr. Martin looked at me quizzically.

"Calf's too big to come out," I informed him. "But it's alive and pretty strong right now. If we want to save it, we'll have to do a C-section."

Mr. Martin glanced around as if searching for something, holding the rope firmly in his two knotty old hands.

"I can tie her off to the tractor," he said helpfully. "That way I'll be able to help you git that calf out."

Few of these old ranchers seemed to consider what went into delivery by C-section. To do major surgery in field conditions that defied any concession to sanitation was ridiculous. I pretended to mull over his offering.

"Mr. Martin," I said, shaking my head sadly, "we're going to have to get her to the clinic. It's too wet and dirty out here to think we can do the surgery here. I know your trailer's in the shop, but can you borrow one to bring her into town?"

I watched the thought processes turn over in Mr. Martin's head. After a few moments, he nodded.

"Ben Gerick lets me use his trailer sometimes," he said. "I'll call him."

"Good." I turned to the cow. "Let's get her up and to the gate, at least. If she stays on her feet, it'll slow down the contractions a little so maybe the calf won't die before we can do the surgery."

He nodded his agreement, and we coaxed the tired heifer to her chest, then to her feet. I was amazed that she was able to get up at all. She walked, spraddle-legged, down the muddy road before us, as we urged her around the tractor and my truck, toward the gate. At the high ground near the gate, Mr. Martin tied the rope to one of the posts that felt the most securely seated in the wet ground. As long as she was standing up, the cow did not appear to be straining as much. That was good. Mr. Martin went back for his tractor and I for my pickup, and we both left down the mud road. I would prepare for the surgery in the dry cleanliness and relative warmth of my clinic's barn, and he would enlist some help and borrow a trailer to haul the suffering cow. Mr. Martin figured it would take him about an hour-and-a-half to get to the clinic.

At the clinic, I informed my crew what was going to be happening in the next couple of hours. We rescheduled afternoon appointments and prepared for the surgery. A space heater cranked out a small measure of warmth into the chilly barn where the chutes and pens were set up and waiting for the patient. My instrument packs, gloves, and supplies were at the ready. We waited. And waited.

Two hours and Mr. Martin and the cow still hadn't appeared. I had my receptionist call the Martin house. His wife informed us she had not seen him in two hours, not since he had come in and told her he was going with Ben Gerick, Franklin Grief, and Lawrence Brown to get the cow with Ben's trailer. I clicked off the names in my head. I knew Ben Gerick and Franklin Grief. Both were elderly gentlemen like Mr. Martin, retired long years from their careers, spending their time tending their small herds of cows and waiting for their social security checks to come in. I didn't know Mr. Brown, but my guess was that he was of the same generation. I worried about these old men, out in the cold, misting rain, standing in water while trying to load a reluctant cow into a strange trailer. Though she was small, 500 pounds of cow resisting arrest was trouble. After fretting about the situation for another hour, I decided to go out to the ranch and see what was happening.

As I approached the ranch gate, I could see there were two vehicles, as well as Mr. Martin's old tractor, on the lane inside the pasture. One of the pickups had a fourteen-foot stock trailer hitched to it. The only relatively dry spot left to park was on the county road, so I stopped, got out of my truck, and worked my way, rubber-booted, through the slick mud to the pasture. Mr. Martin came around the vehicles to greet me.

They had managed to back the trailer into the pasture so that it was as close as possible to where the cow had been left tied. Behind the trailer stood Mr. Martin's three friends. Mr. Brown was just as I suspected, another senior citizen, rubber-booted, wearing a tattered old coat and a toboggan cap pulled down over his ears against the weather. All four of the elderly gents looked cold, wet, and tired.

The cow was still tied, but now the rope ran from her head through the trailer and out one side, where Mr. Grief held the end, keeping the rope taut. The cow was squatting on her rump, her feet braced in front of her. She wanted no part of the trailer. Around her on the ground lay some logging chains, each probably thirty feet in length. A broken rope dangled from the trailer. I could feel the hair on the nape of my neck rise, even under my wool cap. This had been going on for three hours? This poor cow had been struggling against these ropes and chains and determined old men for three hours? I wondered how in the world her calf could still be alive through that. I wondered how this under-weight, pregnant cow could still be resisting her capture after three long hours. As I stood numb, taking in the story the scene told me, Mr. Martin spoke up.

"We tried pulling her with the tractor, but the rope broke," he said, indicating the frazzled end of a rope dangling from the trailer. "We tried making a come-along around her butt with the chain, but that didn't work none either. We tried a hot shot, but all that did was make her mad."

He paused to let that information sink into my mind. "We was fixing to try pushing her in with the tractor," he finished.

Mr. Brown, a tall, pot-bellied, balding man well into his eighties, coughed from his position on the other side of the cow.

"What we need ..." he said, hooking his thumbs into the belt loops of his sagging pants and hitching them upward, "what we need is a couple more men to help us get her in."

"That's it!" agreed Mr. Grief immediately. "With two more men, we can pick this cow up and set her right in the trailer!"

My mind quickly generated a motion picture of six old geezers in ragged winter gear hoisting up this wet, tired cow, three on each side, and racing with her into the trailer. Six old men yelling "Hut, hut, hut!" in unison as they bore the wretched beast rapidly along. I must have been getting a little too cold and tired, too. Again, I shook my head to clear the image.

I had moved to stand beside the cow, positioned so I could see into the trailer. I tried to see what looked so terrifying to the cow that she preferred struggling against ropes and chains and old men, rather than step up into the only dry area around. Nothing was there. I looked down at the cow. She was squatting down hard against the rope, with fine, white foam forming around her muzzle, her eyes bulging from the effort of resistance. As I looked pityingly down at her, she rolled her eyes up to meet mine.

"Yep, two more men, and maybe some more chain," intoned one of the old men.

I shook my head in sorrow for the cow. I leaned over her slightly and whispered to her *sotto voce*.

"It would be best if you just got in the trailer," I urged her, "before they bring in reinforcements."

The heifer's eyes grew a little larger, and suddenly she stood up, so abruptly that Mr. Grief, on the other end of the suddenly slack rope, stumbled backwards and lost his grip. The cow continued to look directly at me and I at her. She turned her head, faced into the trailer, pitched her ears forward, and snuffled at the trailer floor for a couple of seconds. Then graciously, with all the dignity she could muster, she stepped up onto the trailer floor.

For a few seconds, the creak of the trailer floor as the cow moved forward into the conveyance resonated against the stunned silence of the shocked men. I was just as stunned as they were. Then, coming awake, I slapped my jaw shut, stepped back, and swung the tailgate closed.

Mr. Martin was staring, open-mouthed, at the cow standing quietly in the trailer.

"Let's go," I suggested, acting as though this had been a totally anticipated outcome, exactly what I had expected to happen. All four men suddenly jumped into action, picking up their chains, securing the trailer tailgate, running as fast as their old bones could carry them to their vehicles for the drive to town. I hustled to my own truck, did a careful U-turn on the muddy surface of the road, and led the caravan to the clinic.

❖

It was a successful surgery. The calf, unbelievably, was still alive, vigorous and strong. The cow, her ventral abdomen sporting a row of neat sutures, stood up almost immediately after the surgery. Once released from her restraints, she lowed to her calf and washed it tip to toe. Both of them recovered fully and left for their home ranch after forty-eight hours in the clinic.

Mr. Martin and his cronies still talk of me whispering into that heifer's ear, suggesting she stand up and get in the trailer. I don't know why she did what she did, and so dramatically. Maybe it was she felt my empathy and desire to help her. Maybe she was just tired of fighting. Maybe, too, the calf squirmed and caused her to shift her weight enough that she stood up, loosening the pressure of the rope and giving her a chance to make the choice of going into the trailer.

I don't know, but I don't argue with the power that saved a cow and calf that day and allowed four old men to come in out of the rain.

Mr. Mason's Evasive Cow

*It is just like man's vanity and impertinence to call an
animal dumb because it is dumb to his dull perceptions.*
—Mark Twain

It happened more than once, that unexplained but awesome
experience of a cow seeming to read my mind or feel my empathy for her situation so that she was suddenly cooperative with
my efforts to help her.

Mr. Mason was an older rancher who was not a regular client of
mine. With an apologetic tone in his voice, he made it perfectly
clear he was asking for my help only because he couldn't get hold
of his regular vet. I did a lot of emergency call-outs for that reason
and had ceased being offended at being the last choice in the
phone book. Mr. Mason was a gentleman known locally for his
kindness and consideration of others. I told him I would be happy
to help him out of the crisis with his laboring cow. With directions in hand and Barbara, the high school girl working for me
after classes, in the passenger seat of the pickup, I headed out to
the country on that pretty, early-fall day.

The cattle pens on Mr. Mason's ranch were immaculate, the
fences high and strong, the head gate well greased and in perfect
working order. Mr. Mason met us at the gate. The problem was,
the cow wasn't in the pens. She was down, lying out in the field.

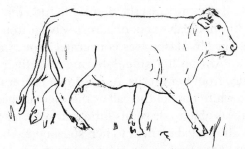

The rancher explained that he had been unable to get her up. There was one small calf hoof showing from her vulva, he said, but she had not progressed in the labor in the previous two hours. She was an older cow and had calved many times before. He knew she was in trouble and was worried about losing both her and her calf.

He led the way on his four-wheeler; Barbara and I followed him across the pasture in my Dodge pickup outfitted with a vet box carrying all the supplies and equipment I might need. Mr. Mason raised Red Brangus, large, deep-red cattle of good size, with long ears and loose skin. The Brahman breeding in his cows was evident, and he said they were good mama cows.

Unfortunately, coyotes and feral dogs had been raiding the local herds and killing calves. In defense of his calves, Mr. Mason kept a male donkey with the herd. The donkey did a great job of guarding the calves from marauding dogs and hungry coyotes. However, the donkey was also leery of people and kept the cows moving away from any humans who did not match his idea of acceptable. The donkey regarded the old rancher on his four-wheeler kindly. My red pickup was another story, in the donkey's mind, and he turned to his charges and hustled his adopted herd away into the trees.

Mr. Mason's property was beautiful. His large pastures were dotted with some of the tallest, straightest pine trees in Houston County. They were so tall, their lowest branches were at least twenty feet up, and the sun easily reached the grass under the trees' canopies. There was very little brush or weeds. It was easy to keep track of the cattle, as the donkey herded the twenty-five or so cows with their calves out of harm's way far from my deadly pickup. The cow Mr. Mason was concerned about was left lying in the open, down on her side, laboring to deliver a calf that wouldn't budge from her uterus. As we drove nearer the cow, we could see the white hoof of the calf at the vaginal opening.

Mr. Mason was able to drive his little four-wheeler right to the cow's side. As he pulled up next to her, she stopped her straining and sat up on her chest in what is known as the sternal position. I was disappointed to see the cow didn't have a rope on her head or around her neck. Cows have a way of being able to leap up and run, even with a calf wedged in their pelvic canal. I've seen them move with surprising speed while in the throes of heavy labor. I've even seen one leap a five-foot fence like a gazelle, a halfway-born calf dangling behind her.

I much preferred to arrive at a ranch with the cow already penned or at least securely tied to something stout. Evidently, Mr. Mason had assumed his cow wouldn't be able to get up and had not taken my advice to put a rope on her before I got there. I hoped she wasn't going to jump to her feet and leave as he fumbled with the lariat he'd brought along with him, but it was too late. The cow spotted my truck. She came to full alert and stumbled to her feet.

The foot of the calf she was trying to deliver disappeared into her depths. Mr. Mason tried to flip the rope over her head, but she easily tossed it aside, watching my truck with pronounced trepidation. She turned suddenly and took off for the rest of the herd that was quickly heading for the outer reaches of the pasture.

I drove over to where the rancher stood with his empty lariat. We conferred. Mr. Mason was positive he could bring the entire group of cows around the edge of the pasture and to the pens, where we could separate out the cow in trouble and deliver the calf. Mr. Mason was an elderly man, gentle and easy in his manner. His concern for the cow was great.

"I don't want the cow to suffer anymore," he said. "This won't take long."

He cranked his four-wheeler and took off toward the herd. True to his plans, the cows circled the edge of the pasture and headed in the direction of the pens, the target cow somehow gamely keeping up. The donkey, however, was worried about strangers in the pasture and had other plans for his herd. Once within sight of the pens, he commenced to drive the cows away from the suspected danger. Using teeth and hooves, his ears flat to his head, he drove the group of cattle past the pens and back into the safety of the pasture. We could do nothing, as the main group of cows headed back into the pasture, our patient doing her best to keep up.

We conferred again. Mr. Mason said he could get the donkey out of there, so we could handle the herd without its interference. He had a small bucket of grain on his four-wheeler and drove out to try to lure the donkey within his reach. While the donkey took the bait, Mr. Mason slid a rope over its head. He then tied the little donkey firmly to a tree. The cows, now without their guardian, should have been easier to herd.

They were not. For whatever reason, not one of those cows would go near the pens. Every time we got them close, one of them would spook and take off, trailing two, three, and finally all the rest of the cows. We abandoned our vehicles and tried herding the cows on foot. We fanned out across the pasture, attempting to haze the herd toward the pens. It was no use. It appeared that one old man, a teenage girl, and a female veterinarian were no match for a group of cattle determined not to be penned. The target cow was fatiguing, and labor was forcing her to slow appreciably. Finally, she stopped and lay down while the other cows drifted away from her.

Mr. Mason again tried to approach her with the rope, but she was wise to him and his motives now. She lumbered to her feet and trotted away. I was no cowboy; throwing a lariat was not on my meager list of skills. I tried, though, but there was no doubt that the cow would remain safe from me. Barbara had done a little roping in her high school rodeo club and thought she might be able to get a rope over the cow's head. The trick would be to get close enough to the cow to make throwing a loop an option.

The cow had given up trying to keep up with her herd mates. Nonetheless, it was obvious that she was determined not to be roped. She was equally determined not to be hazed into the pens. She was walking slowly, lying down when she got some distance from us, jumping up when we got near, and then doubling back on us toward the pasture, over and over. After about the sixth attempt to pen her, Mr. Mason called me over for another conference. We'd been chasing the cow for close to two hours. Evening was falling. At this point the cow was heading away from the pens, and it was a clear shot to the pasture in front of her. Our chances of catching her looked pretty hopeless. She stopped to grunt and strain against a contraction, the calf's one foot making an appearance before once again sliding out of view.

"I can't stand to see her suffer," Mr. Mason told me. "It looks like we're not going to catch her. The calf's probably dead by now anyway. I'm going to go back to the house, get my gun, and put her out of her misery. You ladies might as well go on home."

The three of us stood quietly watching the cow as she strained a little and moved a bit farther away. She was obviously in distress. I hated to see an animal suffer, but I hated even more seeing one die needlessly. If we could get her in the pen, I felt confident I could reposition the calf so the cow could deliver normally. However, if the owner didn't feel that we were going to catch her, I couldn't justify my time in chasing her either. Nonetheless, I felt badly for the cow as well as the owner.

"I sure hate for you to lose a good cow like that," I said, shaking my head sadly. I felt my heart go out to the cow as she stumbled farther away from us. Suddenly she stopped and swung her big head towards us, both ears angled forward as if to hear every last syllable we spoke. Her big, dark eyes regarded us for a moment, nostrils flaring with her labored breath. She looked back toward the disappearing tails of the rest of the herd. After another moment, she turned and stared off toward the cattle pens behind us. With what appeared to be purposeful determination, she began to walk, then struck out at a fast trot, circling around us.

"She's heading for the pens!" Mr. Mason exclaimed in surprise. He ran for his four-wheeler, while Barbara and I scrambled for the pickup we had abandoned earlier to pursue the cow on foot.

The cow disappeared between the tall trees. I was afraid she would be headed back around the edge of the field when we drove out of the trees toward the pens, but ... no! There she was, still making a beeline for the pens.

Unbelievably, she trotted right through the gates of the pens. Mr. Mason drove up behind her and shut the gates. The cow trotted through the maze of pens and entered the long chute, undirected by any of us. She slowed to a walk and moved down the chute all the way to the head gate. We were flabbergasted, but hurried to shut the gates and put the poles behind her, in case she changed her mind and decided she had to leave. But she showed no indication she was going to try to get away. When she reached the end of the chute, she stopped and stood quietly at the head gate.

We were so relieved to have caught her and so amazed at the way it had happened, we could think of nothing to say to one another. Rather than catching her head, we put a pole behind her butt so she couldn't back up. I got my water and soap, pulled on the long, plastic OB gloves, and did a quick check of the unborn calf's position. It was not a huge calf, but his head and one leg were turned back into the cow, locked behind her pelvis, preventing his birth. Because the cow had been up and moving most of the time, she had not been able to strain so much that she wedged the calf into too tight a position. Mr. Mason had found her before she had lost too much amniotic fluid and before the uterus had contracted tight around the calf. I had room in the cow to work.

I quickly set to righting what was wrong. I had no sooner maneuvered the calf's head and leg into the proper position than the cow gave a mighty heave, grunting with the effort. The calf practically shot out of the cow. Barbara and I caught him and eased him to the ground. He was alive. He shook his head vigorously and began to bawl in indignation over his rude arrival. The cow answered her calf with a soft, low hum. We carried the calf out into a pen and laid him down, where he continued to snort and take in deep breaths. I did a quick check of the cow for problems, and finding none, we released her from the chute. She immediately trotted over to her newborn, lowing continuously, and began to lick and clean the shiny, dark-mahogany bull calf.

It was an extremely satisfying piece of work. Mr. Mason was very grateful and happy that we were able to save both his good cow and her calf. To this day, I am in awe of the cow's sudden awareness of her impending fate and her surprising decision to abandon completely her plan for escape and head for the cattle pens.

She knew, somehow, that we were her only salvation.

Country Dogs

Lots of people talk to animals.
Not that many listen though. That's the problem.
—Piglet

It was an amazing thing to me that an animal could sense a person wanting to help it, as did Mr. Mason's cow. It was an overwhelming feeling, to receive that gift of trust from a creature whose only instinct is to run for safety when pain is at the front of its thoughts. But to have that happen in reverse, to be the one needing empathy and help, and to have an animal or, in this case, several animals seek to help me was utterly humbling.

Cows are certainly not the only animals I've had read my mind, understand my intent, or otherwise seem to know exactly what I'm up to. In my practice I worked with cats, dogs, and horses, as well as cattle. I have a strong connection with cats, and many people brought their feline pets to me, knowing the cats would be treated with dignity and respect.

Dogs that were patients or boarders in our clinic were usually calm and easy to work with, and many appeared genuinely happy to come into the building and visit with us. However, the same dogs that were submissive and trusting at the clinic could behave in an entirely different way while on their home turf—defensive of their territory and aggressive toward visitors.

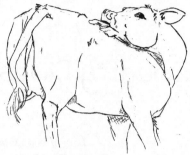

Sometimes on ranch calls I had to wait for the owner to tie up or cage a dog who took offense to my presence, much like they did to mail carriers or meter readers. I understood where the dog was coming from, though, and rarely had a problem with one after it was established in the dog's mind that the owner welcomed my visit. Subsequent calls to a ranch were usually peaceful. But I would not get out of my pickup on a property with a dog baying its warning. The night I nearly walked into a pack of guard dogs was one I won't soon forget.

When Mr. Lloyd called one fall day, it was already dark. We had just switched back from daylight savings time to standard time. He said he'd penned up a cow at noon, because he was sure she was going to calve any time. When he'd gotten off from his job, he'd gone out to check the cow.

"She had the calf, Doc," he informed me. "He's okay, but the cow prolapsed. Everything came out. I never seen one that big."

"Is she standing up?" I asked. A prolapsed uterus is a life-threatening situation for the cow. The longer the everted uterus stays outside the body, the greater the chance it will be damaged by trauma or impaired circulation.

"She's up," Mr. Lloyd replied. "She's nursed the calf, too. I don't want to lose her, Doc. She's a gentle thing. She's a young cow, too."

"Give me directions to your place," I said, snatching a pen and note pad off the desk. He gave me directions using landmarks and mileage, as the county roads were poorly marked and tended to look the same in the dark. I felt I could find the place, though, and headed for my truck.

It was a crisp, cool autumn night. No moon or stars showed through the cloud cover, and the darkness was total. In the country there are no streetlights and no businesses lining the roads, casting illumination over everything. Traffic tends to be sparse after nightfall, too. I headed north out of Crockett, and about ten miles out of town, the white sign that read "Patterson Cemetery Road" loomed out of the dark on the side of the highway. Following the directions given me, I turned left off the paved highway onto the well-tended dirt road.

It seemed that most of the back roads in Houston County were named after either a cemetery or a small country church. There were an impressive number of these cemeteries and churches in the county. Some of them dated to the 1800s. Slow to change, Houston County officials had bucked the statewide trend to change from named to numbered roads. Makeshift signs still pointed down various back roads with such names as "Shiloh Primitive Baptist Church Road" and "Everett's Cemetery Road." The roads kept their traditional names, even when the churches had fallen down and disappeared and the cemeteries were so overgrown with weeds as to be invisible. I had been down Patterson Cemetery Road before and had never seen the cemetery.

With no moon or stars in the sky and without the lights of homes, stores, and other vehicles, the blackness of the night was complete, except for my truck's headlights on the narrow road in front of me. It would be very hard to find the turnoffs ahead.

The directions said to drive four miles down Patterson Cemetery Road and look for a fork, where I was to take a narrower, unmarked road to the left. In about a quarter mile, I would see a set of board-fence pens just inside a pasture. Mr. Lloyd would be waiting in his pickup at the gate.

After three miles, I slowed my speed to lessen the chance of missing the turnoff. At four miles, I didn't seen a fork in the road. I crawled along, searching the dark for some break in the brushy growth that might indicate a road. Another half mile and a dirt road branched off to the left. It was not exactly a fork in the road but more like a lane coming in from the left. I kept on the main road a couple of hundred yards farther and passed a house with lights blazing and a couple of pickups and cars in the yard.

I drove slowly for another half of a mile. By now I was five miles from the highway, a mile past where Mr. Lloyd said the turn would be. Frustrated, I made a U-turn in the road and back-tracked to the house and the lane that had forked off to the left. I turned down that dirt lane.

The house's lights disappeared behind me as I drove along the very narrow lane. The roadside weeds and brush were so close to my truck I could almost reach out the window and touch them. This sure didn't look like the right road. I decided to find a place to turn around and go back toward the highway, feeling I'd missed the proper turn after all.

The lane did not widen and no side roads appeared out of the gloom. The lane took a decidedly steep, downward pitch. The roadbed appeared to be turning to sand, and I struggled to keep my truck moving.

I must have traveled at least a quarter mile when ahead of me in the dark loomed a shiny aluminum gate, sixteen feet wide. The weeds encroached upon the road right up to the gateposts. Great. No way to turn around. I'd have to back out.

I put the truck in reverse and eased my foot onto the accelerator, as I looked over my right shoulder out the rear window. The truck's tires caught and then slipped, spinning in the sand. The incline of the road was so steep and the sand so slippery and loose that if I continued to press the accelerator, I would cause the tires to dig great troughs and bury the axle. Shoot, I said, or words to that effect.

I put the truck in neutral, found my flashlight, and got out. I checked the left rear tire. Not quite to the axle, but getting there. I turned the flashlight beam to the gate, hoping it was unlocked so I could drive into the pasture and make a U-turn and drive out the lane, but a chain with a padlock encircled the latch end of the gate and the post. The padlock was secured. I kicked the ground in frustration. My truck rumbled in sympathy.

At that time, I didn't have a cell phone or a two-way radio with which to call for help. I got back into the cab, put the truck in reverse, and tried to back out again. This time the tires spun madly, flinging sand out from beneath them and settling the truck deeper into the troughs. I cut off the engine, got out, and turned my flashlight beam under the truck to inspect the axle. What axle? It was buried, with the truck into sand up to the rear bumper.

Frustrated, I squawked an unkind word at the world. It echoed in the stillness of the night. I turned off the flashlight. Man, it was dark. I quickly snapped the light on again.

I'd have to walk back to the house I'd passed before turning down the lane. Mr. Lloyd had given me a cell phone number to call, if I got lost. I was lost, all right. Perhaps I'd be able to use the phone at that house to call Mr. Lloyd and let him know where I was and why I was delayed. I locked the truck, buttoned my coat, and started up the steep, sandy lane, flashlight in hand. It was a bit steeper than I realized. Shining the flashlight back toward my pickup, all I could see was the tailgate and the reflections of the taillights. I trudged on.

The lights of the house came into view as I topped the hill and the lane leveled out. I was about 100 yards from the house. I counted two pickups and a car in the yard. That seemed like a lot of vehicles; maybe they were having a party. I didn't intend to do more than ask for the use of their phone. Hopefully, it wouldn't be a problem.

As I stepped into the yard, still 100 feet from the house, a dog barked, one quick, cautious, canine "Who goes there?" A big dog, too, from the sound of it. I stopped in my tracks, a slight feeling of anxiety coming over me.

Here I was, trespassing on some dog's territory in the middle of the night, with nothing but a flashlight to defend myself. I waited to see what the dog would do. I moved my flashlight beam, to let the animal know where I was. An outline of a dog appeared, silhouetted against the house lights. It was facing me, at full alert. It had the outline of a rottweiler, a big, beefy dog, its massive head held high and a short tail erect and stiff. Oh, great. The evening just kept getting better and better.

"Hello!" I called, hoping I sounded friendly to the dog, hoping the dog had alerted someone inside the house who would come out to investigate if the dog barked again and maybe save my life.

The sound of my voice caused the dog to erupt into a frenzy of deep-throated baying barks, which in turn apparently alerted an entire pack of dogs, all of which joined the first dog in a frenzy of defensive, warning, foaming-at-the-mouth barking.

I stepped back. There was no way I would be able to outrun a pack of dogs, even if I'd been wearing track shoes instead of the knee-high rubber boots I had on. In front of me the silhouettes of a dozen dogs suddenly loomed up against the house lights, a dozen huge dogs with cropped tails and big heads. Frightened, I backed up another step. This maneuver only served to encourage the dogs to jump toward me, baying and bellowing at the top of their lungs.

There was nothing I could do. When I did not move, the dogs held their ground and continued to fill the night air with deafening roars. If I backed up, they advanced on me. It was safer for me to stay put and wait, hoping the residents of the house would respond to their guard dogs' howls and come check on what was disturbing them.

No one came to the door of the house. The dogs continued to keep me in one place, all of them in a line at the edge of the light thrown from the porch. They did not step into the shadows where I stood, but they did not cease their barking and baying.

What was the matter with those people? Were they deaf? I couldn't hear any sound coming from the house, such as music or a loud television. I could certainly hear the dogs and I was sure anyone in the house could hear them also. I was sure the entire county could hear the dogs.

I couldn't shift a foot without the middle dog getting excited and lunging forward, his barks exploding louder and more threatening. If I froze in place, he would stop his advance and slow down his barking.

I realized after a moment that the dog in the middle was the biggest dog, and most probably a rottweiller. However, I had to admit the dogs that ranged out to his side were smaller. Maybe not a dozen, either, but there were still at least six of them, all raising Cain and facing me head on, their tails straight up over their backs.

One had to be a dachshund, yapping so enthusiastically that each soprano vocalization caused his short front legs to pop off the ground. Another appeared to have the build of a border collie, and he would slink from one end of the line of dogs to the other to issue a rapid-fire bark at me and then pace back to the other end to repeat the warning. A short, thick dog next to the biggest dog had the outline of a bulldog, and I was sure it was his deep, gruff, intermittent bark that acted as the bass in this canine concerto. A couple of the other dogs registered as generic brands, maybe a little hound in them from the tone of their barks. All of them barked continuously and furiously. No one in the house was responding to the barrage of barking. I didn't know what to do.

Now I was getting a little annoyed at being held in place while no one bothered to come to the door to check on the racket. Unable to move an inch and frustrated with my feeling of helplessness, I whined out loud without meaning to. The effect of my voice on the dogs was immediate and startling. They hushed as one. Absolute quiet descended again on the night air. Surprised at the dogs' response, I waited, watching their silhouettes before I cautiously tried another keening whimper. The dogs were motionless, each head cocked to one side, registering my plea.

"I'm lost and cold and tired," I whined piteously. "I have to get to Mr. Lloyd's cow and help her. My truck is stuck in the sand."

Every dog's head shifted abruptly, cocking in the opposite direction. They were listening. I felt encouraged.

"I need help," I wheedled sadly, slumping my shoulders in despair.

The dogs were nothing but outlines, but I could see what they were doing. Still at attention, heads cocked at me, they started to wag their tails in short, "we hear you" movements. Even the rottweiller's tail, though short, jerked back and forth in response to my plea. I whined again, no words, just a high-pitched, frustrated moan.

The rottweiller ducked his head, twisted his whole body downward to the ground, and came toward me, wiggling all over. I didn't move. He slithered up, grinning up at me. The other dogs approached also, surrounding the rott and me, all of them mimicking his posture. I was being accepted as okay, it appeared. It seemed as if they were inviting me to come on up to the house. Encouraged, I started across the lawn, the half dozen dogs fawning around, licking my hand, and ingratiating themselves to me. I was emboldened. I strode up to the house, murmuring thanks to the dogs, patting the heads that bumped my hand, and smiling at them as they escorted me to the back door.

At the door, all the dogs sat down, calmly watching me, waiting for me to do whatever I needed to do next. I peered through the window of the storm door, on through the glass panel in the wood door. I could see children's school knapsacks lined up against one wall of the hallway beyond the door, but no person was within sight.

I rapped on the glass of the storm door. Before my knuckle tapped the glass a second time, a frenzied, high yipping erupted from inside the house. Another dog, a small one, leapt into view through the glass. It was a Yorkshire terrier, and it kept leaping wildly up to look through the window in the door, yipping shrilly, before falling out of view again. I glanced at the dogs surrounding me. Each and every one of them grinned happily, tongues out, ignoring the yipping of the Yorkshire. Their demeanor told me it was all right to try knocking on the door again. I rapped the glass three or four times.

All my knocking seemed to do was inspire the Yorkshire to higher leaps and sharper yips. If there was a person inside the house, they did not respond to the dog's noise or the tapping on the glass. I looked down at the rottweiller. He was staring intently at the doorknob.

"Should I open the door?" I asked him. He opened his huge mouth and laughed up at me.

I tried the storm door. It was unlocked. It opened outward, and I swung it open. The Yorkshire went ballistic as I tapped on the glass panel in the wooden door. I called out a loud "Hello!" Strangely, no one answered.

This was very weird. I looked around the yard. With all those vehicles, why wasn't anyone answering the door? The dogs waited expectantly. I tested the doorknob. It was unlocked. I pushed the door open.

The Yorkshire went into a panic, yipping so rapidly I wondered how he could draw breath. He turned and scurried down the hall as fast as his short legs could carry him. I stepped into the entrance hall and yodeled another "Hello!" Nothing. No one answered.

I was getting very nervous about the whole situation. I took a couple steps into the house, closing the door carefully behind me. The little dog suddenly lost his nerve and fled again. He never stopped yipping, though.

I looked down at my boots, covered in sand and mud, and slipped out of them, not wishing to leave tracks on the clean tile floor. The room up ahead and to the left was brightly lit. I called out again as I eased toward the room. Still no one answered.

I sneaked a peek around the end of the wall. It was a kitchen/dining room. A table stood in front of me, and beyond that a service bar separated the dining area from the kitchen. The table was set with dinnerware, flatware, and glasses with place settings for ten people. A large basket of garlic bread, half empty, sat in the middle of the table. Spaghetti and meatballs had been served to each plate, and half of the food had been eaten before the diners had apparently dropped their forks and left the table. This was very odd. I called out again; there was no answer. The only sound was the frantic yipping of the little terrier from a room on the other side of the house.

There was a tabletop phone at the end of the counter in the kitchen. I tiptoed across the room in my stocking feet. Now I could see the entire kitchen. A big pot sat on the stove; a bowl half filled with salad and a plate of chocolate chip cookies were on the far end of the counter. The cookies looked good. I considered trying one, but decided it was best not to tamper with the evidence.

I picked up the receiver of the phone and listened for a dial tone. Phew, there was one. I pulled out the piece of paper with Mr. Lloyd's cell phone number and quickly dialed. Mr. Lloyd answered before the phone had rung twice.

"Hello?" he said, a little anxiety in his voice.

"Mr. Lloyd, this is Dr. Cooper-Chase," I said. "I'm lost. I got my truck stuck in the sand on a little road that dead-ends at a pasture gate. I'm using the phone in a house, but no one is here, so I don't know who lives here. I guess I missed the fork I was supposed to take."

I knew I was talking rapidly, nervously. I glanced around the unnaturally quiet room. Even the little house dog had quit yipping.

"You're in a house?" Mr. Lloyd asked. "There's no house where you're supposed to be."

"I know that," I replied, feeling just a little bit exasperated. "I think I passed the place I was supposed to turn. I'm about four-and-a-half miles down Patterson Cemetery Road. This house is brick with white trim. They have about six or seven dogs here."

I told him my story and described the dirt lane where I'd got my truck stuck. Mr. Lloyd was silent.

"Mr. Lloyd?" I queried, wondering if I'd lost the connection.

"Wait!" he said suddenly. "I know where you are! I'll be there in about ten minutes!"

He hung up before I could say another word, before I could give him the number of the phone I was using, before I could look around the kitchen for something with the family's name on it. I hung up the phone. Well, if he didn't show up in ten minutes, I'd call him again.

I really did wonder where the family was who lived in the house, the family who had jumped up from their dinner and left, leaving the house unlocked and an assortment of vehicles parked in the yard. What was going on?

I left the dining area and went back to the entrance hall. The Yorkshire had crept out of the room he had taken refuge in, and when I emerged from the dining room, he erupted into a yipping fit again and dodged back the way he'd come. I followed him into the next room, which frightened him and caused him to retreat farther into the house.

The living room had a nice lived-in look but was empty of people. I followed the sound of the little dog's yips across the room into a narrow hallway. Doors opened on either side, presumably into bedrooms. Dare I look? What would I see if I looked? I was scared to look and scared not to look. I eased into the hallway and peeked into the first open door.

The Yorkshire had hidden under the bed in that room, and he dodged under the bed skirt as I peered around the door. There was no person in there. A quick glance in the other doors revealed a bathroom, another small bedroom, and the master bedroom. All the rooms were devoid of people. I hurried back to the entrance hall, pulled on my boots, and eased open the door to the outside.

All the dogs were on the porch, waiting for me to reappear. They seemed genuinely happy to see me again, greeting me with licking and joyful bouncing around. They escorted me to the edge of the yard, as I walked out to the lane to wait for Mr. Lloyd, but they did not leave the boundary of the lights of the house. I continued on the lane. The dogs waited on the lawn of their home, once again silhouetted against the light.

From down the road came a set of headlights and the rumble of a big truck engine. The dogs remained silent until the vehicle turned onto the lane, and then they began a barrage of barking that would have sent any stranger running. I spoke to them softly, telling them it was okay and that I knew who this was. Remarkably, they hushed. I flashed the beam of the flashlight to show the driver of the truck where I stood. The dogs remained quiet, watching, as the truck pulled up next to me and stopped. It was

Mr. Lloyd. I was never so happy to see someone as I was to see him. We exchanged hellos.

"Where's your truck?" Mr. Lloyd asked. I pointed down the lane.

"It's pretty steep and sandy," I said. "I don't know how we'll get it out of there."

"This truck will pull it out," he informed me confidently, patting his truck's door fondly. "I got about 100 foot of chain in the back. I'll hook it to your truck, and I'll drive down only as close as I need to and hook my truck to the chain."

It sounded like a plan to me. We drove down the lane, parked, and pulled the heavy chain out of his pickup. I could see the dogs pacing the yard and wondered if they would start barking again or come down to where we were. They did neither. They seemed to understand they had no jurisdiction that far from the house.

Mr. Lloyd got the chain on the ball hitch of my truck, and we lined the chain out along the ground toward his truck. He had tow hooks installed on the front of his truck, a huge one-ton dually work truck. I sure hoped it wouldn't grind a trough beneath each of those double wheels and bury his axle, too.

"You get in your pickup, put it in neutral, take the brake off, and just steer enough to keep it straight on the road," Mr. Lloyd said. I nodded my understanding and trotted to my truck and got in. He strode to his truck, got in, cranked the big engine, and began backing up slowly, taking the slack out of the chain. I felt my pickup jerk. Mr. Lloyd's truck howled and inched backward, spewing sand with the four big rear tires. I prayed he would not get stuck too. We didn't move. My pickup dropped back into its ruts as Mr. Lloyd eased up, put his truck in neutral, and got out. I met him halfway.

"Start your engine," he said. "You're pretty stuck there. It's going to take both engines to get you out of there. Ease it back as I pull, okay?"

"Okay," I agreed. We went back to our respective vehicles.

This time, when Mr. Lloyd's truck had taken the slack out of the chain and begun to haul back, I eased down on the accelerator and off the clutch. There was a moment of worry as the tires spun without gaining purchase, and then the truck lurched out of the rut. Mr. Lloyd's truck backed up the hill, easily dragging my pickup. He didn't stop until we got to level, solid ground.

After removing the chain, I told Mr. Lloyd to lead the way to his cow. He nodded and headed out. I looked over to the quiet dogs and saluted them.

"Thank you!" I said meaningfully. The silhouettes wagged their tails in acknowledgment. I got in my truck and took off after the receding taillights.

❖

About half a mile down the main road, Mr. Lloyd made a sharp right turn off the Patterson Cemetery Road. This was the fork I had missed in the dark. I followed him down the dirt road about a quarter of a mile and into the pasture where the cow pens were.

In a pen stood a black Brangus cow, invisible in the moonless, starless night, but revealed to us in our flashlight beams. A dark-brown, newborn calf was curled up at her feet. The cow blew her breath sharply at us.

"She's usually a real quiet cow," Mr. Lloyd said. "She's a little upset right now."

"Can't blame her," I said, shining my flashlight down her length. A large, irregular, dark-red blob was suspended from her rear end. It was definitely a prolapse and definitely the entire uterus. However, with what I could tell from her behavior, we still had a good chance of saving the cow.

Mr. Lloyd went into the pen, cautious enough of the cow to stay near the fence, and shushed at her, causing her to move away from him and toward the alleyway at the end of the pen. She walked quietly down the chute to the head gate, where we trapped her quickly. I went back to my truck for supplies.

❖

A prolapse of the uterus is a very scary thing to see, especially to the uninformed. Mr. Lloyd had done the right thing by penning the cow and keeping her quiet until he got some help.

Normally the uterus begins a process called "involution" right after the calf and afterbirth have been delivered. During the calf's development, the uterus expands and enlarges from its pre-pregnancy size of about eight inches in length to an organ large and strong enough to contain a fully developed calf of from fifty to eighty pounds. Added to that is, of course, the placenta and all the fluids that go with the job of growing and sheltering the calf in utero. Amazingly the involution process will shrink the entire uterus down to nearly the original size within forty-eight hours after delivery.

A prolapse of the uterus may occur after a difficult or prolonged delivery of a calf. Pain will cause the cow to continue to strain after the calf has been born. With the cervix wide open, the organ can turn inside out, coming out of the cow. If the blood supply is not interrupted, involution will still occur, although the organ usually cannot reduce fully while still inside-out on the outside of the cow. If the blood return from the uterus to the body is interrupted, then the uterus cannot shrink and will often continue to get larger. There is a grave danger of the cow injuring the uterus in her attempt to get up and move around, with hemorrhaging and death occurring. Some cows continue to strain due to the pain of the prolapse, causing their intestinal organs to prolapse also.

Luckily, this cow was calm and not had injured the everted organ. By flashlight illumination, I gave the cow an epidural in her sacral-coccygeal space. This would prevent her from straining against my efforts to replace the exposed uterus and relieve her pain until the involution process had gotten under way.

If a prolapse is not tended soon after its occurence, the involution process causes the cervix to constrict, making the return of the uterus to its home difficult and maybe impossible. Happily, this cow's cervix was still open.

As I worked, I asked Mr. Lloyd about the family whose house I had trespassed into to get to the phone.

"You know, I don't know," he answered. "I've seen the kids and all those dogs, but I don't know their name."

"Where were they?" I asked, as I cleaned up the brick-red uterus with a mild soap and water. "There was no one home, except the dogs. And all those vehicles in the yard. What happened to them?"

Mr. Lloyd appeared to dwell on the question.

"I bet I know," he finally said, smiling with his voice out of the dark. "They have kids, right?"

"Right," I said, starting the process of easing the prolapsed uterus back into its rightful place. "Looked like grade school, from the book bags in the hallway."

He chuckled. "I'll bet the other vehicles belong to other parents with kids. I'll bet you a dime to a dollar they all sat down to dinner and had to get up and run off to a ball game or something. I know the mother drives a minivan. Bet they all piled into it and took off—kids, parents, and all. Everyone except the dogs."

It sounded likely. "I checked the bedrooms," I confessed. "No dead bodies anywhere. You're probably right."

I finished with the cow. She was a little wobbly in the rear from the epidural, but once released from the chute, she made her way back to her calf, where she eased herself to the ground to rest. I was sure she'd be all right.

I cleaned up my equipment and stowed it in the truck. Mr. Lloyd got out his checkbook.

"Tell you what," he said. "When I come down here in the morning to check on this cow, I'll stop over and check on that family, too. It's about time I introduced myself to them; we are neighbors, after all. I'll call your office, let you know what I find out."

"That would be wonderful," I said gratefully. "It was sure a spooky thing, going in a house like that and everything set for dinner, the food half eaten, and no one there. Real scary."

Mr. Lloyd did call me the next morning to tell me he'd stopped in to meet his neighbors, the Hopewells. There were the parents, two grade-school-age children, and seven dogs. He said the dogs wouldn't let him out of his truck, and Mrs. Hopewell had to leave the house and walk out to his truck to see what he wanted. Nice people, he said, but fierce dogs, every one of them. The rottweiller could sure bark, but he was most worried about the ankle-biting dachshund and never did get out of his truck while there. He did not tell her I had gone into the house to use the phone; he didn't want to worry her with that detail.

❖

Mr. Lloyd's cow recovered and raised her calf with no further problems. There was little that was routine about that particular call-out. I'll never forget that pack of dogs and the way they allowed me onto their territory and into their home that dark night. I thought about it many times in the years that followed.

It had to be another case of the ability of animals to read the true intent of a human being, but also of the powers that be once again helping me out of a fix.

Part 2

Unhappy Cattle

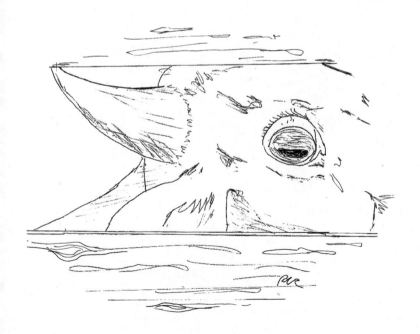

Mr. Swanson's Lame Bull

Animals can communicate quite well. And they do.
And generally speaking, they are ignored.
—Alice Walker

Unlike dogs, which are often credited with high intelligence by their people, cows are often thought of as mindless creatures whose job it is to graze, give milk, and supply meat for steaks and hamburgers. While they do graze, give milk, and most of them do eventually end up as protein on our dinner plates, cows are far from mindless. Every cow, bull, or steer has its own personality, its own take on the world.

One of the things I learned while dealing with cattle is how to read body language a little bit better, that of both cattle and people. Cattle are experts at reading the body language of humans, whether or not most humans are aware of it. Cattle are, after all, prey animals and, as such, must be constantly aware of every little movement in their surroundings. The size of the animal doesn't matter. Grown bulls can be just as leery of strangers as are smaller cows or calves. They do not wish to provide humans with a meal any sooner than they absolutely have to, either.

❖

A call one morning came from a rancher whose cows I'd seen a couple of times. The pens and chutes on this particular ranch

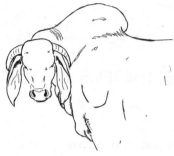

were very poorly designed and constructed of faulty materials. When I saw chutes like that, my immediate inclination was to rope the cow and work with her tied to a tree or stout post, rather than chance her smashing through the frail pens to freedom.

This time, the rancher had a bull with a lame foot. Knowing, as I did, the condition of his chutes, I suggested he might want to bring the bull to the clinic, rather than have me come to his ranch. Mr. Swanson assured me that the bull in question was gentle, having been halter-broke as a calf, and would lead like a puppy on a string. So, with doubts, I agreed to drive out to see the bull on his home turf.

The first thing I noted on arrival at the ranch was that the pens were shabbier than I remembered. To really draw attention to their dilapidated state, in the crowding chute was an enormous gray Brahman bull. The hump on his back cleared the top board of the sagging fence by what looked like three feet. He had an enormous head, upon which sat huge, swept-back horns above thick, heavy brows that almost obliterated his tiny eyes. He had his left rear foot cocked and delicately balanced on the toe, indicating pain in that foot. I got out of my truck and stood by the relative safety of its red bulk, watching the bull with great trepidation.

Mr. Swanson came out of his house and crossed the yard to the pens. He was a small man, probably in his late 60s or early 70s, and wheezing from emphysema. He was attempting to untangle a small, ratty rope that didn't look like it could restrain a Chihuahua. I hoped he didn't intend to rope the bull with it. Mr. Swanson coughed once or twice into his handkerchief and pointed to the swollen rear leg of the bull.

"Been like that about three days," he said. "He's pretty lame."

That much was obvious. I was going to have to look closely at the foot to determine the reason for the pain and swelling. That meant restraining the bull in some manner. I sure didn't like the condition of the pens, though, especially with such a big bull.

"I can walk up to him," Mr. Swanson said. "He's real gentle. He's used to being handled."

However, I noticed that Mr. Swanson did not move to approach the bull but stood next to me, fiddling with the sorry little rope in his hands.

"We'd better see if he'll go down the chute," I said. "I will probably have to pick up his foot to look for a nail or something else stuck in it."

"Looks like foot rot to me," Mr. Swanson offered. "Maybe you can just give me something to squirt on the foot."

"We have to look, first," I replied. "It won't do any good to put something on the outside, if there's a nail inside." Mr. Swanson shrugged as if in partial agreement.

We held our positions, shuffling from foot to foot for a few seconds longer as we eyed the bull. It looked like it was going to be me who would have to suggest to the bull he needed to go down the rickety chute. With great reluctance, I slid over to the corral fence.

There was no way the sagging fence was going to hold me while I climbed it. The gate was made of barbed wire and tied shut with an assortment of baling wire, hay string, and a little bit of spit. I decided I was going to have to separate the wires and crawl through the loose wire fence. So I did.

When I straightened up on the inside of the pen, the bull was still standing stock still, the wounded foot cocked ever so slightly. He was staring over the fence toward his cows in the pasture. I wondered if he would jump the fence or, because of his hurt foot, simply smash through the flimsy barrier and head out to pasture. I took a step toward him.

He swung his massive head around to his flank and fixed his bright little beady eyes on my wide, suddenly very frightened eyes. He dropped his head a notch, never moving his eyes from mine, and blew out his nostrils—a long, loud, and promising exhalation of breath. He wasn't going to move, and he had requested, in not-so-subtle bovine language, that I keep my distance. I swallowed. Could I bluff a lame bull, especially a 2,000-pound lame bull, into moving away from me? I took a half a step toward him.

While my foot was still suspended in mid-stride, the bull did a half turn on the forehand, swinging his huge body around to face me head on, flicked his tail once, so the switch of it lay over his hip, and dropped his head just one iota lower. Then he raised a forefoot and with his massive cloven hoof, slowly drew a line in the dirt of the pen.

I can take a hint. With barely a falter, I swung my advanced foot back behind me, and took a step backwards. The bull unhurriedly shook his head at me, causing a loop of saliva to slowly flip up over his muzzle. I took another cautious step back, keeping my eye on the bull. Satisfied that his message was received, the bull raised his head, eyed me carefully to be sure I was retreating, and turned away. He flipped his long ears back in the direction of the pasture, watching the cows.

I crawled out of the pen, unhooking the fence barbs from my clothing as I struggled through the rusty barbed wire, and stood up, shaking slightly, next to Mr. Swanson.

"I don't think I'm going to be able to look at his foot," I said, pointlessly. Mr. Swanson smiled gently.

"Tell you what we'll do," I continued, hemming a little as I cleared my throat. "I'll leave a squirt bottle with some medicine in it. If you can get next to the bull, like you say you can, try putting a little on the foot, between the claws, twice a day and see if that helps. If it doesn't, you might have to get him in a trailer and bring him to the clinic."

Mr. Swanson nodded in agreement. I rummaged around in the truck, found the medicine I was searching for, and handed the bottle to him. With just a moment of hesitation, he went back to the pen and crawled through the wire. I was afraid to watch. He walked slowly up to where his bull stood facing the pasture. The bull appeared to be ignoring the slight human being coming up on his side. Mr. Swanson patted the bull firmly on its massive left shoulder. The bull flicked his left ear backwards at him, once. Mr. Swanson loosened the nozzle of the bottle, took careful aim, and squeezed the bottle, sending a stream of liquid toward the wounded rear foot of the bull. The animal stepped sideways from the man, swung his head toward him, snorted in annoyance, and returned his gaze to the cows in the distance. I was astonished.

Three days later Mr. Swanson called to tell me the bull was no longer lame. Apparently, it had been a mild case of foot rot and not a nail that had caused the lameness. Nevertheless, the bull's acceptance of his familiar owner's presence and the way he allowed him to medicate that very sore foot was what amazed me.

It Could Have Been Rabies

There is no fundamental difference between man and the higher
animals in their mental faculties. … The lower animals, like man,
manifestly feel pleasure and pain, happiness and misery.
—Charles Darwin

Just because you try to handle every cow with gentleness and respect doesn't always mean the cow will respond in kind. A cow that has been brutalized in the past might have a hard time accepting a change in handling technique. A cow under the influence of a disease process might also have a hard time understanding much. For instance, a condition commonly known as "grass tetany" affects a cow's ability to handle stress.

Grass tetany is caused by a magnesium deficiency. It is seen during certain seasons of the year, and its development depends on certain weather conditions, as well as feed intake. Also called "grass staggers," a cow with the disease shows signs that include lack of coordination, irritability, and convulsions. She might appear to forget who her usual handler is and be hypersensitive, belligerent, and defensive. She may be fighty, may bellow and charge, and if she's able to keep her feet under herself, might knock down and gore whoever comes near her.

❖

I had such a case one fall day. Mr. Edwards, the rancher who called on me, was relatively new to the business of keeping cattle.

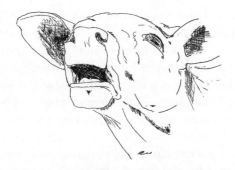

He had a cow acting odd, he said. She was a nice young cow, one he had raised from a calf, and one who would eat from his hand and enjoyed having her neck scratched. Now she was trying to fight, he said, and had frothy white saliva dripping from her mouth. He was alarmed by his normally placid cow's belligerent behavior and was worried that the cow might have rabies.

Although rabies is always a possibility in any warm-blooded animal, in this case I believed grass tetany was the most likely cause of the cow's sudden change of behavior, based on the recent weather conditions we'd had and the quality of the forage that was available. I suggested to Mr. Edwards that he stay away from the cow and not aggravate her. Let me get a look at her first, I told him.

Luckily for all parties involved, the cow had staggered into a good pipe corral and fallen, giving Mr. Edwards time to close the gate on her. When I arrived at the ranch, the cow, a large black Brangus type, was in the pen lying near a sizable mud puddle, her eyes wide and unblinking, her head trembling, and slobber trailing from her mouth. When she heard our voices as we surveyed her from the safe side of the fence, her head whipped around in our direction, and she sucked her mouth open and emitted a quavering bawl. The trembling of her head increased as she tried to keep her eyes focused on us. She attempted to lunge to her feet, gained them shakily, and charged at us, bellowing and slinging slobber. Mr. Edwards and I stepped back from the pipe fence, thankful for the two-inch iron rails between the cow and us.

If ever a cow displayed all the symptoms of rabies, this one did. She looked for all the world like the cow in the old black-and-white film we were shown in veterinary school of a cow gone mad from the rabies virus. While that disease was on the list of possible diagnoses that I named off for the owner, grass tetany was still number one on my list of causes for her behavior. Bearing in mind that a brain-addled cow was a brain-addled cow and was capable of doing grievous bodily harm, regardless of what was addling her brain, my next dilemma was how to restrain the cow for treatment purposes.

Getting the cow to come in close enough to rope was not going to be the problem. She was practically crawling up the fence to get to us. She had no horns; therefore I'd have to rope her around the neck. As she bellowed and flung her wobbling body at us one more time, I dropped my lariat noose around her neck and took a wrap of the rope around a post in front of the cow and another wrap about ten feet down the rail, out of harm's way of the cow, and tied it off.

Now the cow was seriously angry. I had to get a halter on the fighting cow quickly so I could loosen the rope on her neck, which was threatening to strangle her. Mr. Edwards was nervous and inexperienced in dealing with such fury in a cow. I was able to get the halter on her in record time and without injury, which was quite the trick with this cow so intent on hurting me. Once the halter was in place, I tied the halter rope up high on the fence and loosened the neck rope.

All this time, Mr. Edwards was standing back from the action, wringing his hands, his eyes huge and staring in disbelief at his formerly gentle cow. He was thoroughly convinced that rabies was the sure-enough cause of this behavior. I still didn't consider rabies as the number-one diagnosis and was fervently praying I was right.

Once the rope was secure, the cow became still, glaring at me as I perched on the fence's top rail. She was trembling from nose to tail, her tail whipping back and forth in fury. I had to decide next on how to dose her with a remedy to counteract the hypomagnesium state I hoped she was in.

The standard treatment for an active case of grass tetany was an intravenous solution containing the magnesium along with the other minerals of calcium, phosphorous, and potassium. However, I couldn't see myself getting cozy enough with this cow to try to get a three-inch-long, 14-gauge needle into her jugular vein. I liked living too much.

A recent development in veterinary medical treatments at that time was an oral paste containing all the minerals the intravenous product contained. Its intended use was for mild cases where the patient was cooperative and easily restrained. This cow was not on the label.

Looking at my enraged patient, I hesitated only for a moment before deciding to try the paste. It would be a lot easier and safer to inject a paste into this cow's mouth than to crawl in beside her to give an IV. Maybe it would work well enough to take the edge off the cow's condition so I could then place an IV later. After locating it in my truck, I placed the large cylindrical tube of paste into a dispenser gun and cautiously climbed back up on the top rail of the fence, so that I was once again above the securely tied cow.

Upon seeing me lean out over the fence, the cow bellowed loudly, her mouth wide open as she lunged toward me. I put faith in the fence to hold me and in the rope to hold the cow, and I aimed the tip of the paste gun into the gaping pink mouth and fired, rapidly squeezing the trigger and effectively dumping the entire contents of the tube into the cow's oral cavity. I dropped down and jumped back from the fence. The cow was cursing me from her side of the fence and flinging herself from side to side. I withdrew to stand next to Mr. Edwards, who stood a safe distance back from the fence and the furious cow.

"I'm not sure if this will work," I said. "It might take awhile."

"What if she's got rabies?" asked the rancher, casting a sidelong glance at me while keeping his main focus on the agitated cow.

I pondered the question. I wasn't at all sure how long she'd live after beginning this display of symptoms, if it was the deadly virus acting on her mental workings.

"She'll die," I said. "But I don't know how long it will take. Maybe a couple of days."

We stood solemnly, studying the cow.

"If it is rabies," Mr. Edwards asked, "what do we do after she dies?"

I slowly wiped some cow slobber off my hands. I had been exposed to rabies once before, while working as a technician, and had had to take the full series of fourteen shots—twelve of them in the belly—to prevent infection. Though the treatment had changed over the years, it was still no picnic to have to endure. If contracted, a rabies infection was inevitably fatal, however, and there was no real option other than the preventative injections if exposure to the virus had occurred.

"First we'd have to take a brain tissue sample and have it checked for rabies," I told the man, and in my mind's eye I saw the brutal procedure of removing an animal's brain. With a large animal such as a cow, such a job is butchery at its worst. I did not look forward to it.

"If she tests positive," I continued, "the state will get involved with the quarantine and vaccination process for you and the animals that have been pastured with her."

Mr. Edwards groaned out loud. I could tell he regretted having called a veterinarian out to see the sick cow. A thought suddenly occurred to me. I turned to him.

"Are you worried about getting rabies from her?" I asked. "Because to get it you have to have been bitten or otherwise have exposure to her saliva." I studied the man carefully. He shifted his weight nervously and cast worried eyes in my direction.

"Did she bite you?" I was wondering how he put himself in a position to get bitten by a cow.

"She didn't attack me, if that's what you mean," Mr. Edwards said. "I thought maybe she had a stick in her mouth because she was foaming so much and wouldn't take any cubes from me." He gestured weakly toward the cow. "She wasn't so upset then, not acting so … crazy. So I reached in her mouth, looking for a stick. She kind of bit me."

He pulled off the left glove of the pair of leather gloves he wore, grimacing as he did so, and showed me the hand it had enclosed. I winced when I saw the crushed index finger, still raw from the trauma caused by the cow's molars. It sure looked painful.

I mulled the information over. Having a human exposed to a possibly rabid animal made this a lot more serious case. I was debating whether to euthanize the cow right then and there and send her brain off for testing, when I noticed a change in the rancher's position. He was leaning forward, intently watching the cow through the pipe rails. The look of consternation on his face had changed, becoming one of wonderment.

"Doc?" he asked softly. "Does that cow look quieter to you?" I followed the rancher's gaze through the pipe fence to the cow.

And, indeed, she did look better. She was no longer trembling. Her tail was still, except for an occasional swipe at flies. Her eyes, protruding and showing the whites in her fury at us earlier, had settled peacefully into their sockets, allowing the lids to close and hide the white portion of the eyeball and giving her that gentle, bovine look once again.

"If it were rabies, she wouldn't get better from the medicine," I told Mr. Edwards. "Let's see what she does when we go up to her."

He held his ground only long enough for me to get a head start. We approached the cow, as close as the fence would allow. The cow watched us benignly. She rolled her tongue up over her nose, snorted gently, and regarded us kindly.

"I think the medicine worked," I said carefully. "It was grass tetany. She's going to be all right."

The change in the cow was like night and day. She was once again the gentle black mama cow the rancher had raised from a calf. However, rabies being the strange, unpredictable disease that it is, I stopped Mr. Edwards as he reached out to stroke the cow's head.

"Let's do this," I said. "Let's take off the halter but leave her in the pen for ten days. If she gets sick again, we'll be able to treat her more easily. If she dies, we'll have to check her brain for rabies."

The man withdrew his hand from the cow's head hastily. It sounded like a plan to him.

I climbed up on the fence and reached over, tentatively testing the cow's response to my approach. She snuffled my hand, ears forward and interested, eyes calm and quiet. I loosened the halter quickly and slid it off her head. The cow gave a quick fling of her head, turned away, ambled to the water trough, and drank, long and deeply. I heard Mr. Edwards heave a mighty sigh of relief.

"That's a good sign, isn't it?" he asked hopefully. "Her drinkin' water like that."

"Excellent sign," I said, also encouraged by seeing the formerly deranged cow behaving with grace and dignity. "An excellent sign."

❖

It was unquestionably the most rapid and dramatic response to treatment of grass tetany I had ever seen. The cow did not relapse into her former state of illness and, with proper feed and mineral supplements, returned to her normal self. Ten days later the owner released a fit, healthy cow back into his pasture.

The Cow with the Very Sharp Horns

Holy cow!
—Harry Caray

Since so many diseases that affect the brain can cause the same array of symptoms, it's often a challenge to come up with the real reason for an animal's altered behavior. Besides viral infections such as rabies, there can be bacterial diseases or chemical imbalances like grass tetany. Anything causing a high fever can cause symptoms of dementia, resulting in a normally placid beast going on a rampage. Fred Porter's cow was such a case, and she very nearly was the last cow I would ever examine.

❖

Mr. Porter called my office one beautiful autumn Saturday seeking help for a problem with a cow. The Porters had a weekend ranch in Pennington, a small town about twenty-five miles from Crockett. Weekenders, as we called the folks who lived elsewhere and visited their ranches on weekends and holidays, comprised a substantial number of my clientele, and I was always happy to help them out. The Porters were among my favorites.

"She must have had her calf last weekend," Mr. Porter reported to me. "We live in Dallas and only come down on weekends, as

49

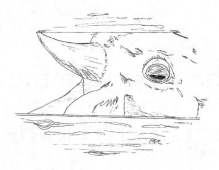

you know. She's an older cow, and she's had lots of calves. She was in labor when we left last weekend, but we didn't worry about her. But today she's looking bad. She's acting a little crazy, and she's lost a lot of weight. Looks like afterbirth or something hanging out of her. We found the calf. He's alive, but he's pretty puny, like he hasn't nursed much."

I told him I'd be along directly. My assistant, Leslie, wanted to go with me on the call. She was a good hand, so I told her to jump in the pickup. Off we went to the little township of Pennington to see Mr. Porter's sick cow.

When we arrived at the modest ranch, Mr. Porter had the cow in his good board pen. The pen was muddy from the past week's rains, and the cow had churned up the ground in the enclosure considerably while going around and around, seeking to escape. She was thin compared to the other cows out in the pasture. The cow had her head up, her eyes showed white, and she was snorting loudly through her distended nostrils as she ran along the fence line. She stank badly from the rotting rope of what appeared to be afterbirth dangling from her vagina. Her udder was flabby and did not appear to be producing milk. The calf was lying down in another pen, separated from the cow, which paid him no mind as she sought to escape.

We checked on the calf first. He was still alive, but obviously undernourished and weak. My guess was the cow was running a fever from the infection caused by the retained afterbirth. Fever will cause a serious reduction in milk production, as well as weight loss. The calf was simply not getting enough nourishment from his sick mother. We had to get the cow cleaned up, the afterbirth removed, and antibiotics administered. Once her fever was down and the infection was under control, the cow would be able to resume producing milk for her calf.

The first trick, though, was getting the cow into the chute and restrained in the head gate so I could work on her in relative safety. Besides being a little crazed from the fever she undoubtedly had, what made this cow particularly tricky to work with were her horns. Each horn was easily eighteen inches in length and curved forward from her head. They had wickedly pointed tips that almost twinkled in the afternoon sun. The cow knew, exactly to the millimeter, the length of each of those horns. She raked them along the fence as she trotted back and forth, shook them menacingly at us as we neared the fence, and otherwise indicated she was well aware of the weaponry she carried on her head. She knew she had us intimidated.

Most cattle operations have a large gathering corral, into which the cows are herded from the pasture. From this corral, the cows can be directed into a smaller crowding pen, usually attached to a chute. The chute directs the cattle to a head gate, in which the cows are caught around the neck, to restrain them for whatever procedure is necessary, be it branding, vaccinations, deworming, or other medical treatment.

This cow did not want to enter the crowding pen. Each time she circled the larger corral, she'd veer away from the entrance to the smaller pen. The big, twelve-foot gate was wide open, but she refused to go through it. I was worried the cow would overheat or otherwise stress herself if she continued to careen around the corral.

My mission was to save the cow and along with her, the calf. The cow didn't understand why she was cornered, in pain, and separated from her calf. She only knew she wanted out of the corral. There was nothing I could do for her until I could get my hands on her, however. She had to go into the crowding pen and down that chute to the head gate.

Mr. Porter had long, lightweight bamboo poles to help direct cattle in the pens from the relative safety of the top board of the surrounding fence. He and I climbed up the sides of the fence and attempted to use the long poles to steer the cow toward the crowding pen. The cow simply tossed the poles aside with a flick of her horns and continued to charge around the corral. At one point, she tossed her head and caught the nice, long pole I had in my hand, causing it to fly away, into the center of the muddy corral where it stuck, straight up, in the wet ground.

It was a good, stout pole. I wanted it back.

As the cow charged to the other end of the corral, I slipped down the fence boards into the corral. My booted feet sank six inches into the mud. Leslie and Mr. Porter warned me to be careful. I was fairly young, fairly agile, and fairly stupid. I didn't see a problem with what I was doing. I waded through the mud toward the pole.

As I bent to pick it up, I saw the cow throw her head in my direction. She snorted loudly, dropped her horned head, and charged across the corral toward me, the mud making loud sucking noises as it pulled at her cloven feet, slowing her advance somewhat. I turned to run to the fence, confident I would make it with time to spare. However, the same mud that slowed the cow down also had a firm grip on my rubber boots. A thrill of panic shot up my spine as I fought to pull my feet loose from the mud. One foot slid out of its boot, as I got a hand on the board fence. I tried to pull the other boot loose, Leslie and Mr. Porter hollering at me to hurry up.

I was suddenly in a time warp. Things were moving slowly—the emergence of one foot from the stuck boot, my hands grabbing for the fence, and my attempt to climb while one boot, with foot, remained firmly stuck in the mud. Everything was slow except the charge of the cow. In a split second she was upon me, bawling, flinging saliva from her mouth, her head down and those twinkling horns aimed right for the small of my back.

I twisted around to face the oncoming cow, one foot on the fence, the other foot in its boot, still firmly planted in the mud.

I could hear both Leslie and Mr. Porter screaming, as they reached for me from the other side of the fence. All I could see, though, was that approaching cow, those wicked horns leveled at my midsection.

I was going to die. On this pretty fall day, in a muddy cow pen, I was going to die from being gored in the belly by a sick cow. I couldn't get my foot out of its mud-trapped boot so I could climb the fence to safety. I turned completely around to face my executioner, my back to the fence.

And that cow hit, hard, her head centered right on my abdomen. The board fence behind me shuddered from the impact. I was screaming or, at least, I was emitting a high-pitched whine, waiting for the pain. I wondered why I couldn't feel the horns. It must have been the adrenalin surging through my system. The cow bellowed, her breath hot on my legs. I looked down at her, expecting to see blood gushing from around a horn stuck in my belly.

What I saw was the top of the cow's head centered on my navel. She had hit the fence with her horns so hard—one on each side of my waist—that the horns had embedded in the wood, holding her fast. I was alive and unharmed but trapped between the fence and cow's forehead, a horn on each side of my waist.

I felt like I was in a cartoon, but with none of the humor. My ears seemed to be stuffed with cotton. Through it I could hear Mr. Porter and Leslie screaming. I realized I was screaming too, above the bellowing of the angry, fevered cow whose hot breath burned my thighs, her body twisting as she pushed angrily toward me and tried to do me grievous harm. The board at my back vibrated from the shaking the cow was giving it, first pushing toward me, then pulling back, as she tried to free her horns.

I knew if I was going to stay in one piece, if I was going to live, I had to get up the fence and away from the cow. I couldn't turn around, as the fit between the fence and the cow's head was tight. I tried unsuccessfully to lever myself up between her horns, one hand on each horn. The cow tried to pull back, but she was stuck tight in the board. She flung her body from one side to the other, bellowing with rage. The board cracked but still held her tight for the moment.

I began to pound her on the poll of her head with my fist but all that did was make her angrier. I began to punch her nose with my right knee, bringing my leg up as hard as I could, over and over again. After about the third punch, it was evident to me the cow was trying to pull away, but her horns were still stuck solidly in the boards behind me. I stopped thumping her nose with my knee. Panting from fear and exertion, I twisted my body at the waist just a little and somehow pulled myself up the railing, leaving the cow in the board and my boots in the mud.

I scrambled to the top of the fence just as the board splintered and the cow pulled herself free. She blew and hooked her horns upwards toward me a couple of times before trotting off to the other end of the corral. I was panting as though I had run a fifty-mile race at full tilt. Leslie and Mr. Porter were excitedly asking me if I was all right and checking to see if the cow had hurt me. They were on both sides of me, patting my back and checking for blood.

"No, I'm fine," I assured them two or three times.

As my breathing slowed and nerves calmed, the cottony sensation in my ears dispelled, and I became aware of how frightened Leslie and Mr. Porter were from the looks on their faces, by their own scared, panting breaths. I turned to see where the cow was.

"Good Lord, girl," Mr. Porter commented, an audible tremble in his voice. "I wasn't sure you were going to get out of there."

"Neither was I," I concurred. "My boots are wrecked, though. And I didn't get my stick back, either. It was a good stick, too."

Mr. Porter snorted a nervous laugh.

"Well," he said, "you sure can keep your sense of humor."

What else could I do? There was no reason to get angry at the cow—she couldn't help how she was feeling. She stood at the other end of the pen, snorting and pawing the ground in frustration, before she began her mad trot around the corral again. This time, however, instead of bypassing the gate to the crowding pen, she ran through it. As she entered the smaller space, I jumped down, bootless, into the muddy corral to swing the gate shut behind her. She hooked at it once as it swung toward her but didn't attempt to escape.

I retrieved my ruined boots and pulled them back on. They were cold and uncomfortable from the mud inside. I didn't have another pair with me, so they would have to do. I looked around and saw the pole the cow had knocked from my hand. I pulled it from the mud, certain I would need it again.

The cow, once confined in the smaller pen, seemed to accept her capture. She calmed down and dropped her head, and her respiration slowed. With a little coaxing, she trotted into the chute leading to the head gate. As she stuck her head out the opening of the head gate, Mr. Porter deftly caught her. We would now be able to work on her. With Leslie's help, I got my equipment from my truck, hoping the tremors from my scare would subside enough for me to do my work.

The first thing I did was get my thermometer out and take the cow's temperature. It was a burning 105 degrees. Normal for a cow is 101. This was a very sick cow.

The placenta, or afterbirth, was very rotted, smelled horrible, and required me to glove up and go into the cow to loosen it. It fell free from its uterine attachment with just a little effort. We then lavaged her uterus with disinfectant, gave her medication to combat the infection and fever, and turned her out with her calf. Mr. Porter thought he could pen up another nursing cow and get the calf to nurse it until the mother cow was again producing milk.

Leslie and I drove away from the ranch, leaving Mr. Porter to settle the cow in the pen with hay and water. He reported to us later that the cow's fever had disappeared after a couple of hours, and she had calmed down. Her udder filled with milk within twenty-four hours, and she was able to resume nursing her calf.

❖

For me, this was one more unexpected adventure that came with what should have been a routine job and proved to me once again that powers beyond my scope of understanding kept faithful watch on me as I did my duty.

He Swears He Never Touched Her

Compassion for animals is intimately connected with goodness of character; and it may be confidently asserted that he who is cruel to animals cannot be a good man.
—Arthur Schopenhauer

When I first opened my practice, any person calling for help could depend on my swift and eager response to their animal's need. I had to learn the hard way that not all people were appreciative of my willingness to help. They made it difficult for anyone to want to work for them. Leo Grady was one such person.

❖

I'd already taken my shower and was getting ready for bed one Saturday night when the phone rang. Telephones chiming at such a late hour can make any veterinarian quiver with apprehension. I tentatively picked up the receiver and answered the call.

The gruff voice of an older gentleman boomed into my ear.

"I need to talk to the vet!" he shouted.

After confirming that I was indeed the veterinarian and not the veterinarian's wife, I politely asked who was calling. Instead of answering, the man grumbled some remark about women doing

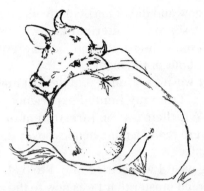

men's work and impatiently asked how much it would cost for me to come deliver a calf. Looking at the clock on the wall, whose hands stood at the ten o'clock hour, I told him there would be an after-hours charge in addition to the regular call charge.

"All you vets care about is money!" He snorted righteously into my ear. I ignored that comment and asked him where the cow was.

"In the pen at my place!" the man almost shouted at me. I held the receiver out from my ear. He had yet to identify himself. Since I still had no idea who was calling, I asked him for that information again.

"Grady! Leo Grady! In Salmon! Up by the Hyle Ranch!" He was shouting now, sounding very agitated.

I was fairly new to the area. I did know where Salmon was, but I'd never heard of the Hyle Ranch.

"The what ranch?" I asked, after writing his name down on my message pad.

"HYLE! The Hyle Ranch! Up near Salmon Lake!"

At this point in my career I had been in Crockett maybe four months. Besides not recognizing the Hyle Ranch name, I did not know who this thundering Leo Grady might be. Here it was 10:00 p.m., and I was on the telephone, a towel wrapped around my wet hair, being yelled at by a total stranger. I didn't like that and considered simply hanging up.

The man certainly gave the impression of being a short-tempered rancher, one who wasn't keen on spending a lot of

money on a cow and didn't particularly like members of my profession. Most seasoned veterinarians will use just about any
excuse to get out of assisting such a client, especially at such an
inconvenient hour of the night.

However, I wasn't seasoned and didn't know if he was as bad
as he seemed. From my limited experience, I did know many
people took out their fear and frustration on the veterinarian,
when they were really feeling helpless over the condition of one
of their animals.

Wondering what I was getting into, I told Mr. Grady in as calm
a voice as I could muster that I was new to the area and not familiar with the Hyle Ranch.

"Well, how much will it cost for you to come out here?" he bellowed irritably again.

By this time I had unfolded the county map and was searching
it for Salmon Lake. I found the little body of water on the map
quickly. I told Mr. Grady the distance to his ranch would determine the cost, along with the after-hours charge. The calf delivery charge would be determined by the time and effort it took to
accomplish the task.

Mr. Grady fumed and sputtered over the line, muttering about
cows not being worth the money spent on them and veterinarians being worth less. I got the impression he might continue in
this vein half the night. I gave him a few minutes to vent his anger
before I finally asked him point blank if he wanted me to come or
not. He stopped his ranting for a moment before reluctantly saying yes, he wanted me to make the call-out. In an irritated and
loud voice, he gave me directions to his ranch.

My husband, Jack, had come into the room while I was still
holding the phone and listening to Mr. Grady's ranting. He'd been
able to hear the man's angry voice and had listened to my end of
the exchange. He knew without asking that I would be going out
that night to a place I'd never been, to face an angry man I had
never met. Without any trouble, he'd picked up on the rancher's
unfriendly nature. He asked me if I wanted him to go along on the
call. I said yes, gratefully.

I got dressed, pinned my freshly washed and still-damp hair up on my head, and covered it with a bandana. I filled a couple gallon jugs with hot water and checked the other supplies in the truck. Map in hand, we headed out into unknown territory.

Mr. Grady's ranch was about fifteen miles from Crockett. The Hyle Ranch sign, a landmark Mr. Grady had given me, was located out by the highway. It was unlit, but it was large and white, and we found it easily enough in the beams of the headlights. I steered the truck down the road next to the sign. As Jack navigated, we weaved along the back roads of north Houston County, looking for a white pickup parked at one of the side roads. Finally, we found the truck, facing up another dirt road.

As we approached, the pickup's door opened, causing its interior lights to come on. A large, big-bellied man, presumably Mr. Grady, climbed out of the seat and walked over to my window as I pulled up behind his truck.

"Took ya long enough to get here!" he snarled, red-faced in the glow of my cab's overhead light. I was taken aback, but before I could comment, he continued barking at me. "We gotta go down this road a bit to get to my pasture. Follow me so you don't get lost again!"

He turned, strode back to his truck, climbed in, and slammed the door to the cab violently.

"What an asshole," my husband observed dryly. "Is that the guy who called?"

"I guess," I answered. "Same voice."

"Why are you going to help him?" Jack asked. "He's a butt."

"He's got a cow in trouble," I shrugged.

Ahead of us, Mr. Grady's truck jerked to a start and roared away up the side road. We followed. After bumping down the dirt lane for a short distance, the pickup turned off the road and jerked to a halt. Mr. Grady got out. Without a backwards glance, he lumbered to a gate, threw it open, climbed back into his truck, and roared into the pasture. Jack and I looked at each other, shrugged, and followed. I stopped inside the gate and Jack jumped out to shut it. By the time Jack got back into his seat,

Mr. Grady's truck had just about disappeared into the dark. Luckily, its white paint and flashing taillights made it a little easier to track in the dark. I was happy Jack was with me. I had no idea what Mr. Grady's behavior would be like when we finally stood face to face.

We were led down a narrow, sandy path into the woods, the trees close on either side of us, until a board cattle pen loomed out of the darkness. The white pickup shuddered to a halt, and the driver emerged again from the vehicle. We pulled up next to him and got out.

"Mr. Grady?" I asked, as I approached the tight-lipped, obviously irritated man. He nodded once, ignoring my extended right hand. After barely acknowledging my introduction to my husband, he jerked his head to the left, toward the pen.

"Heifer's in the pen," he barked. "I found her this morning trying to calve. I put her in this pen, and all I did was watch her all day." His jaw worked, as if ruminating. "Seemed like she wasn't going to have that calf without help, and it was gittin' late. I couldn't get no other vet out here. So I called you. I hope this don't take all night. I want to go home."

I had to wonder to myself why he waited all day to get help. Maybe he'd tried to get some assistance earlier but had dissuaded anyone from coming out with his delightful demeanor. I looked over the high board fence and shined my flashlight beam on the white face of a small red heifer that stood quivering on the other side of the pen. She dropped her head and snorted at me, shaking her little six-inch horns in warning. She looked tired, drawn, and big-bellied.

I scouted out the pen and saw that a high-walled chute ran down the side of the pen on the right. There was no head gate, but I determined we could run the heifer into the chute and put a bar behind her so she couldn't back out. I could examine her safely that way.

When I explained what I wanted to do, Mr. Grady acted put upon. He began grousing about cost again, about the value of the cow, and about all the vets who had refused to answer his earlier calls for help, so that he was stuck with a woman to help him. I could understand why vets familiar with this client might decline to return his calls. I clucked my tongue quietly and went ahead with my work.

The heifer weighed about 500 pounds, a rather small individual to be on the verge of delivering her first calf. I asked what type of bull she was bred to and got back the snapped answer of "red Angus." He delivered a defensive tirade on the bull's suitability to first-time heifers, how none of his other cows had calving problems, and so on and so forth. His tirades were wearing on me. Still, the heifer needed help, so I set to the job.

The heifer was disinclined to enter the chute and seemed determined to exit the pen by any means other than the chute. Thanks to her small size, large girth, and general weakness from a long day in labor, she was unable to climb, crawl, leap, or in any other way make her escape. She finally was enticed down the chute when I dropped down the fence in front of her. She lunged toward me and chased me as I scurried ahead of her down the chute. I made my escape up the inside of the chute and over the top. Jack and Mr. Grady barred her ability to back out of the chute with long wooden posts inserted through the fence behind her. Mr. Grady never once stopped complaining about the expense and work to be done. I ignored him and continued to prepare to examine the heifer.

Because there was no head gate, we had to get a rope halter on the heifer and tie her up. This was accomplished with flashlight illumination and luck. I climbed into the chute behind her, and Jack passed me a gallon of warm water, a couple of OB sleeves, and my disinfectant soap. I did a fast examination of the heifer's uterus.

In a normal calf delivery, the calf presents with its two front feet first with the head following just about even with the calf's knees. With this heifer, I found the calf dead, its two front feet set back behind the cow's pelvis and its head turned backwards. The calf did not feel too large for the heifer; it was just improperly positioned. It was impossible for the cow to deliver without assistance.

Even the little manipulation I did during the exam caused the heifer's legs to buckle. We were going to have to let her back out of the chute so we could tie her to a post in the pen. That way, if she fell during the delivery, which she undoubtedly would, she wouldn't become lodged in the fence, unable to get up again. It would also give me room behind her to do my work.

Mr. Grady continued to complain bitterly about money, as we allowed the heifer to move backwards slowly, careful to keep the rope of the halter tied around a stout post as we went.

I explained to Mr. Grady what was going on with the heifer, how the calf was jammed tightly into the pelvic canal, and how it might require some time and effort to remove. He swore loudly, saying he never had such problems, how he had watched the cow all day but never touched her. He complained how she wasn't worth the trouble and money, amongst other things. I wondered why I was there. Jack glanced at me and shrugged, as if to ask the same thing.

After lubricating my gloved hands and arms, I went in search of the calf's front hooves. Jack, holding the flashlight in one hand and the cow's tail in the other, watched as I carefully reached in and searched around with my fingers. As I moved my hand around in the warm interior of the cow, I felt something a little out of place. Puzzled, I carefully grasped the object and brought it out into the light.

What emerged turned out to be a long orange string. I held it up to the light so Jack could see it. Mr. Grady, griping away, was standing off to one side in the darkness and apparently didn't see the string I had found in the cow's insides. Jack made a knowing face in reaction to my grim smile.

In a loud voice intended to be overheard, he asked, "WHY, IS THAT A HAY STRING YOU FOUND IN THAT COW?"

"I BELIEVE IT *IS* A HAY STRING!" I answered just as loudly, grinning at my husband in amusement.

"NOW, HOW DID A HAY STRING GET INTO THIS COW?" Jack practically bellowed at me.

"WELL, I DON'T KNOW!" I replied, so loudly my vocal cords ached. "BUT THE STRING APPEARS TO BE TIED AROUND THE CALF'S LEG! OH, LOOK! THERE'S ANOTHER STRING ON THE OTHER LEG, TOO."

Mr. Grady grew very still. Without looking in our direction and without another word, he walked away from us, out the gate, and climbed into his truck, slamming the door so the light clicked off and left him in darkness. Jack and I grinned at each other. I went back to work. Obviously, in spite of his protestations to the contrary, Mr. Grady *had* tried to deliver the calf himself by tying hay strings around the legs of the calf to provide some pulling traction. Rather than remove the strings after his own unsuccessful delivery attempt, he had tucked the hay strings into the cow, still attached to the legs of the calf, before calling in desperation for assistance. Had he really believed a veterinarian would not find the hay strings and know that someone had attempted to deliver the calf?

With only the sounds of the cow's grunting breath, the crickets, and the night-bird calls, Jack and I went to work to deliver the dead, wedged-in calf. It required the removal of the calf's head, but once that was done, the rest of the small calf slipped fairly easily from the cow. The heifer was greatly fatigued and lay still, gathering her reserve strength while we cleaned up the equipment, medicated her against infection and pain, and put my tools back in the truck.

As I washed my hands and arms of the smell and fluids from the heifer, Mr. Grady got out of his truck, checkbook in hand. He glanced once at the resting heifer before silently taking a pen from his shirt pocket to write the check. He never offered a comment or indicated any displeasure at the price I quoted. He quickly wrote out the amount I requested and thrust the check at me.

As I wrote the number of the check on his receipt, I told him the cow needed to rest a few minutes more and then we would see if she could stand. I thought it best if she stay in the pen for the night, with fresh water and some hay and feed.

Without acknowledging that he heard my advice, Mr. Grady stuffed his receipt in his pants pocket while walking over to the pen. He opened the gate and approached the heifer. She was still lying down, in sternal position. We had already removed the ropes restraining her.

The cow swung her head back toward her owner, her eyes wide and glowing in the flashlight beam. She suddenly snorted angrily and leapt to her feet with surprising agility and vigor. Mr. Grady stopped cold in his tracks in shock at her reaction to his presence. The cow whipped around to face him, dropped her horn-studded head, and charged.

The overweight rancher whirled around and, in an astonishing burst of speed, took off out of the pen. The heifer was right behind him, her head lowered, the sound of her snorting breath filling the night air. She was so close to him he was unable to swing the gate shut as he made his escape. He headed for his pickup, his big belly leading the way, his legs a blur as they pumped. The enraged heifer hooked her horns toward the seat of his pants. He jumped and, amazingly, was able to hoist himself into the bed of his truck, out of harm's way. The heifer circled the truck, her little horns clanging on its metal sides as she hooked upward at the man, her tail whipping back and forth as she bawled at him in fury.

Jack and I stood frozen in amazement beside our truck, as we watched this mini-circus by flashlight. Having decided her quarry had escaped, the heifer suddenly swung toward us. A chill raced up my spine at the sudden danger. We were so intent on watching the cow chase the man that we'd remained in a highly vulnerable position. We stood stock-still with nowhere to run. The heifer appeared to appraise us carefully, then shook her head and pawed the ground once. Apparently her opinion of us was not the same as the one she held for Mr. Grady, because she did not charge us. She snorted, turned, and trotted off, a slight wobble to her rear end, down the darkened path into the night.

When the clicking of her hoofs on the path had faded in the distance, Mr. Grady carefully climbed down from the bed of his pickup and got into the driver's seat without a word. He cranked the engine and backed his pickup away from the pen. We scurried into our truck and followed him back out the twisting lane through the woods to the main gate. At the gate Mr. Grady pulled to one side and got out to hold the gate for us. I hollered "Goodnight!" as we drove past him, but he neither nodded nor saluted in dismissal.

Not surprisingly, Mr. Grady never called on me again, day or night. I didn't care, really, as his sort made my work harder to do. His check didn't bounce, either, so I was quite satisfied with the outcome of that late Saturday's work.

Part 3

Special Deliveries

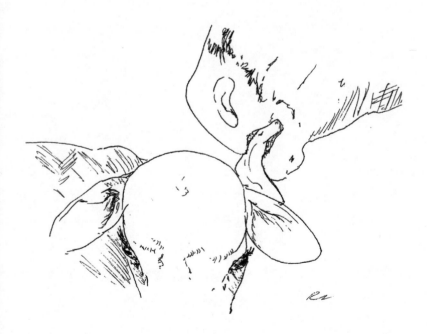

Born Alive!

The greatness of a nation and its moral progress
can be judged by the way its animals are treated.
—Mahatma Gandhi

After going on a few calf deliveries with me, my husband, Jack, was wondering if calves were ever born alive in Houston County. All the deliveries he had witnessed were of dead calves, often putrid by the time veterinary services were called upon. He didn't go on very many cow calls with me, and I had delivered a number of strong, viable calves, so I kept hoping one day he would come along on one that resulted in a calf born alive and healthy.

❖

One afternoon a client, Herbert Weir, called and said his first-time heifer was trying to calve. Nothing was coming out but two feet. The heifer had not been in labor long, he claimed, and he could see the calf's feet wiggling a little. He was afraid the calf would die if not delivered soon and wanted me to come as quickly as possible.

It was a Sunday afternoon, so Jack wasn't at work. I asked him if he wanted to ride along, lend me a hand, and maybe get to see a live-calf delivery. He agreed somewhat reluctantly to give it one more go.

The homestead was far out in the country. We arrived to find the cow, a small but well-fleshed Holstein, in a pen near Mr.

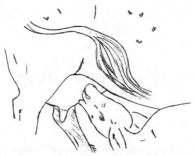

Weir's house. She was standing up and appeared very alert and very unhappy to be penned up away from the other cows. From her vulva protruded two white calf's feet, still draped in the amniotic sac. The calf to which the feet belonged was apparently still alive, as the hooves would jerk and wiggle as the cow shifted around the lot.

We roped and tied the cow to the nearest and safest fence post (not always the same thing on most of the farmsteads I visited). I gloved up while Jack helpfully got hold of the cow's tail to keep it out of my way. The calf was indeed alive with its nose stuck under the brim of the cow's pelvis. With a little manipulation, I was able to bring the muzzle up and get it headed in the right direction. I put a chain on each foreleg, handing one chain handle to Jack while I kept one. We applied a little traction and a robust, black-and-white bull calf easily slithered out of his mama and plopped onto the ground.

Jack was delighted. As I cleaned up my equipment and repacked it into the truck, Jack marveled at the calf's long, wet, floppy ears, the pink tongue sliding in and out of his mouth as the newborn wiped his own nose, his heaving sides as the calf drew in the air of his new and much larger world.

As the calf began to struggle to his feet with the new mother cow lowing and encouraging him with long licks of her rough tongue, Jack crowed with excitement. I was fascinated watching him watch the calf. He insisted on staying at the ranch so he could watch the calf finally gain his unsteady legs and totter to the cow's udder for his first suckle.

Mr. Weir said not a word. As he and I picked up and put away my equipment, I caught him casting a quick glance at Jack now and then. I think he might have viewed Jack as maybe a little eccentric, possibly even a little "touched."

I finished putting away the cleaned equipment and joined Mr. Weir as he stood watching Jack coo over the calf. Mr. Weir couldn't stand it anymore. He leaned over to me and cupped his hand around his mouth.

"Ain't never seen a calf born, has he?" he whispered.

"He's only been on a few calf deliveries with me," I told him. "This is the first live one he's seen."

Mr. Weir drew back and smiled; he nodded in understanding.

"Ah, the live ones," he said. "They're every last one a miracle."

I smiled back in agreement. Miracles indeed.

The Duvalls of Greenfield

We can judge the heart of a man by his treatment of his animals.
                                        —Immanual Kant

Working with cattle meant, of course, working with the people who took care of them. Word of mouth from appreciative clients led to other people calling on my service, and I never hesitated to respond to their calls for help. And so my practice grew.

I came to have the Duvalls as clients by referral. They lived two counties over, near a small town called Greenfield. It was fifty-six miles from the clinic door to the Duvall's barnyard. Since most of my clientele were within thirty miles of the clinic, to have me drive almost twice that distance meant they must have liked my work.

Virtie Duvall's father, Glen Bradley, Sr. (known locally as "Slim"), lived in Houston County and was a regular client of mine. Slim told the Duvalls about me, after hearing Virtie's sad story of cow and calf losses in the preceding months. Apparently, they had called on their local veterinarians on seven different cases of dystocia and had lost the seven cows along with the calves. Slim told them that I'd been able to deliver successfully all the calves he'd called me out to assist into the world. I don't remember if that was true or not, but in comparison with the deaths of seven cow/calf pairs, I must have sounded like a magician.

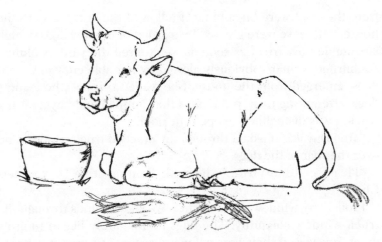

So, Mrs. Duvall called the clinic one cool spring day to ask me to come out and help a two-year-old registered Beefmaster heifer in labor. The thought of losing still another cow to dystocia was unbearable to them.

I truly didn't know what to expect. The Bradleys, my clients, ran a commercial cow operation—cross-bred cows mated to quality bulls to produce good-growing calves for feed yards. The Bradleys' heifers tended to be well developed by the time they were turned in with a bull, and their calving problems were few. However, just because the Duvalls were related to the Bradleys didn't mean they ran the same kind of operation. I wondered what condition the cows might be in. I almost expected to see runty heifers and huge bulls, to account for the deaths of seven cows and their calves.

The Duvalls were well-established ranchers, but if their own veterinarians were unable to help the cows, how would I be able to? At the time, I was young, new to practice, and ready for any challenge, so I agreed to drive the fifty-six miles to see if I could help. I checked my truck for supplies, equipment, and fuel and told my assistant, Leslie, to saddle up and come along.

Due to their excellent directions, we were able to find the Duvall ranch—The Diamond D Ranch—without a single wrong turn down the back roads around Greenfield. The Diamond D pastures were thick with spring grass, and the cows we observed from the road were big and fat. I followed the entry lane to the house, where we were greeted by a group of barking dogs, which surrounded my truck as soon as we entered the yard. A plump, sunburned woman, obviously alerted by her able crew of watchdogs, emerged from the house. She waded through the leaping dogs, attempting to stop the ones that jumped and bayed at my truck. I was disinclined to open the door.

"Mrs. Duvall?" I asked through my cracked truck window and over the roar of the dogs.

"Please call me Virtie," she said. "You must be Dr. Cooper-Chase."

I rolled my window down farther. We shook hands through the truck window solemnly. The dogs immediately began to grow quiet. It was as if they were willing to accept our presence based on Virtie's welcoming handshake.

"Mr. Duvall's at the pens with the heifer," she told me, indicating the white pipe enclosure up the hill a little. "I'll follow you up on my four-wheeler, after I put the dogs up."

She turned and hurried away, whistling and slapping her thighs to call the myriad dogs to her. They all turned from the truck and happily followed her, tails up and wagging, having successfully done their proper duty of alerting against intruders.

I put the truck in gear and followed the sandy path to the pens. Inside the first pen, sitting on an ATV, was an older gentleman who I assumed to be Mr. Duvall. There were no dogs at the cattle pens, so Leslie and I got out of the truck. The man waved me over to where he sat.

I understood immediately why Mr. Duvall had to summon help to deal with calving problems. I was also glad I'd brought my assistant on this call. Though well muscled in his shoulders and arms, Mr. Duvall was paralyzed below the waist. I never discovered the cause of his infirmity, but over the following years, I watched him work cows from his ATV with all the finesse and ability of a cowboy mounted on a champion stock horse.

However, getting off the machine and dealing with an individual case on the ground wasn't possible for Mr. Duvall. I found out later that Virtie was herself a fine cowhand, but reluctant to attempt assisting a cow in dystocia. I also learned they had two sons, although neither one lived in the immediate area. Neither of their two grown daughters had an interest in the cows. So, when they had a problem with the cows, the Duvalls called on professionals. After this call-out, I became their veterinarian, and they willingly paid me to make the long drive to their ranch.

However, this first day I was to help out, they did not know me. They didn't know if I would be any more helpful than the veterinarians in the last seven cases. Mr. Duvall was skeptical, without a doubt. He looked me up and down, trying to judge my capabilities by my appearance. I stood a hand taller than his wife, but weighed probably forty pounds less. I'd seen the look a million times. It was a look that held a little disappointment, a little surprise, and a lot of doubt. I smiled, greeted him cheerfully, shook his hand, and then introduced Leslie to him.

His jaws were working a large wad of chewing tobacco, and a thin brown line of juice dribbled from the corner of his mouth. He spat a long, brown stream into the dust of the lot and indicated the cow lying in the pen before us.

She was a large, well-grown Beefmaster heifer. She sat up on her brisket, facing away from us. Her eyes held a tired, preoccupied look, and as Mr. Duvall explained what the problem was, the cow strained half-heartedly, her back bowing upward. A puddle of fluid, red-tinged, had formed in the dirt under her tail. A thick rope of tissue hung from her vulva and a foul smell permeated the country air. Flies buzzed around her noisily. From these pieces of evidence, before I ever touched the cow, I deduced the calf must already be dead.

"She's been in labor almost two days," Mr. Duvall stated and quickly threw a hand into the air as if to stop me from voicing my outrage. "I called all the vets around here first," he continued. "They all made excuses why they couldn't come out. They've already killed seven of these good heifers. I guess they're sick of us."

He spat again, in disgust, in silent fury. I didn't say a word, waiting for him to go on. His jaw rotated as he ruminated on his chaw. "Slim says you can help us," he finished, sighing in resignation.

I shuffled my feet, a little embarrassed, a little afraid. What had Slim Bradley gotten me into? What had I gotten myself into?

"We need to look at her first, Mr. Duvall," I said. "Can she get up?"

"She tried, but she couldn't last time I tried to get her up," he said, indicating a battery-powered cattle prod leaning up against the fence. "She ain't going nowhere."

I nodded, heading back to my truck for supplies and signaling Leslie to come help. First I would examine the cow and see how the calf was positioned and what condition it was in. Then I would attempt to deliver the calf. From there I would be able to rate the cow's chances of recovery.

I got my long plastic gloves, water, soap, and lubricant and went into the pen. Leslie had produced a lariat into which she built a loop to drop over the cow's head. It was a precaution against the cow getting up and leaving the area. As I've mentioned, too many cows judged unable to get up were known to leap suddenly to their feet and run when the work began in earnest.

The heifer didn't seem to notice us and didn't move as Leslie snugged the rope around her neck. I checked her gum color and eyes, her skin tension and pulse. She appeared to be well hydrated, but obviously stressed. I patted her in sympathy and went to her rear end to do the manual exam of her reproductive tract.

The rope of tissue that hung from her vulva turned out to be a calf's tail, wrapped in a little bit of amniotic sac. It was definitely a breech calf. Further exploration revealed the calf to be wedged tightly into the cow's pelvis and already bloated in death.

I sat back, thinking, then turned to Mr. Duvall, who sat watching me carefully, his chin resting on his hands, folded one over the other on his cane.

"Well?" he asked tiredly.

"Breech," I informed him. "And dead. Real dead. Big calf, too."

"Now you're going to tell me only a C-section will save her!" he bellowed while stamping his cane into the dirt, startling me into drawing away from him. "Damn you vets!"

About this time, Virtie, who had trundled up on her ATV earlier, walked over to Mr. Duvall. She laid a hand on his shoulder.

"Now, Arnold," she crooned soothingly. "Give her a chance to finish." She nodded at me to continue, a small, grim smile on her face.

"The calf is dead already," I said. "We can do a fetotomy; that is, we can dismember the calf and remove it that way. It's a little easier on the cow and will give her a better chance of survival. Plus, it'll mean she might be salvageable as a breeding animal. But that will depend on the damage to her uterus," I concluded. I watched Mr. Duvall's face change as he contemplated what I'd just said.

"No C-section?" he asked.

"Not at this point," I assured him.

"Do what you can," he said, shaking his head sadly at the cow. "She's going to die anyway."

With that vote of confidence, such as it was, I signaled to Leslie to help me get my fetotomy equipment out of the truck.

❖

Fetotomies can be exhausting jobs. First, you must assess the cow's condition to determine if she might be capable of surviving the ordeal. Many things—like the size of the cow, the size of the fetus, and how tightly it is wedged in the birth canal—factor into how long the process will take. Other questions needed answers, such as how long the calf had been dead, what position the calf was lying in, and how damaged the cow's uterus and vagina were. You never know, really, until you go to work on it.

This calf had been dead a while, probably for twenty-four hours or so. Once a calf dies in utero, the body heat of the cow accelerates its decomposition. Normally a very warm 102 degrees, a cow's core body temperature rises with fever, stress, and illness. This is good and this is bad. It's good, because a rotting carcass is easier to dismember and remove than a freshly dead one. It's bad, because the toxins of the decomposing calf poison the cow.

It is a nauseatingly smelly job to deliver a dead calf. The highly lubricating fluids of a normal birth process are long gone, and the watery substance produced by the disintegrating fetus is not slippery in the least. It clings to every piece of fabric it touches, it seeps into the pores of your skin, and its odor lingers for days afterward. It's an odor you, as a veterinarian, tend to acknowledge and ignore. Ignore, that is, until days later when you notice bystanders wrinkling their noses in disgust. Then you rush home and scrub for the hundredth time with every cleaning product in the bathroom and under the kitchen sink. It's a smell you end up waiting to disappear as your body replaces your death-smell-impregnated epidermal cells with fresh, clean cells. It's a smell that never really leaves your aura until calving season has been over for a couple of weeks.

Leslie stood back as far as she could from the cow, ready with equipment, ready to assist, but not before absolutely necessary. She cupped one hand over her mouth and nose as she handed me what I needed. I couldn't blame her at all. I had to kneel behind the sick cow, my nose within a few inches of her rump, as I navigated the crowded birth canal, looking for a way to begin the job of removing the calf from its exhausted mama.

Both of the rear legs of the calf were completely forward in the cow, the toes far out of reach inside the womb. Even with lots of lubricating gel, it was difficult to work my way down to one of the hocks. The cow, tired from her two days of labor, offered only token strains. An epidural was not going to be necessary to work on her.

My first cut was going to be an attempt to remove a rear leg at the hip. It was very important to make a clean cut through the hip to minimize the amount of sharp bone fragments that would be a risk to the delicate lining of the cow's uterus. I would have to first thread a long piece of cutting wire over the front of the calf's thigh and then between the buttocks of the calf. The wire must be positioned as high on the leg and as close to the hip as possible to optimize the removal of that leg.

After a good bit of time spent grunting and sweating and pushing and adding lubricant often, I was able to get the wire where I needed it to be. Leslie helped me thread the fetotome, the part of the tool that would prevent the saw wire from cutting the cow. She positioned herself to begin the sawing action.

With a "ripe" calf, such as this one was, that first cut often releases a gush of fluid from the body of the calf, as well as a large volume of gas, the odor of which was usually ten times more powerful than what was already in the air. I held my breath as Leslie began the cut, as my job was to remain on the ground behind the cow. I had to keep an arm inserted in the cow, guiding the fetotome and holding it in position.

For this I went to graduate school for four years? On these gruesome cases, I could do the work, as long as I kept reminding myself that it was a life-saving procedure for the animal.

I glanced at Mr. Duvall. He sat unmoving on his ATV, his hands still folded over the top of his cane, his chin resting fitfully on them. Virtie had gotten into the seat of the ATV beside him and watched the proceedings worriedly.

Leslie worked the saw rapidly and skillfully, and within a couple of minutes the serrated wire had sliced through the skin and rotting muscle of the thigh, into the soft bone, and out the rest of the leg. With a little juggling, the severed leg was removed from the cow.

The leg was huge with bloat, heavy with fluid. I dragged it a distance from the cow, hoping to lessen the smell and the numbers of flies that had found us. The flies settled greedily on the calf's leg, and I returned to the cow. She had acquired a little life, it seemed. Apparently, removing the massive limb had reduced a good deal of pressure on her pelvic nerves. She shifted her weight forward as if to rise, decided against it, and eased back. She grunted as she strained in labor. The rear end of the calf bulged from her vagina, the extra room made by the removal of the leg allowing it freedom to move outward about six inches. The cow strained again, and a gush of foul liquid flowed to the ground. I waited to see what the cow would do next. She settled down onto her chest again, that far-away look returning to her eyes.

I re-examined her. Without that one leg, the delivery was beginning to look like a possibility. It was pretty nasty behind that cow. As I knelt in the brew of mud and rotting fetal tissue and fluid, I asked Leslie for a new piece of wire and went about the task of threading it around the remaining hind limb.

The second leg was cut as cleanly as the first, and I removed it from the area, leaving it next to its mate to be covered with an increasing number of flies. I batted at a few of the flies that were attracted to the cow. Thank God, it was a cool spring day. If it had been as hot as Texas can get early in the year, the job would have been a lot worse. As it was, things were going more smoothly than I'd anticipated. I confidently knelt behind the cow again, signaling to Leslie to hand me a long calving chain. I would loop the chain around the pelvis, in order to ease the rest of the calf's body out of the cow with the calf puller.

The calf puller, also called a calf jack, was a long metal pole with a ratcheting mechanism, a come-along, at one end. A U-shaped piece of hardware, known as a butt plate, was mounted on the other end. The butt plate fitted below the cow's vulva, at the back of her legs. A strap passed over the hips to keep the plate from slipping down to her hocks.

My calf puller was designed with a spiraling bar as the pole attached to the butt plate. The come-along would travel up the pole as the operator worked the handle, moving the come-along away from the cow. The calf, attached by the chain to the come-along, would be slowly ratcheted from the cow. How much tension was applied during this process was important. Too much, and the cow would be injured or the calf pulled apart before it was removed from the cow. To do it right took a little finesse and a little skill, mixed with a little bit of luck and a little bit of prayer.

Another problem that could occur if the delivery was too fast was a complete prolapse of the uterus from the cow. Never pretty, always life-threatening, a prolapse was a mostly preventable and mostly correctable problem possible during any calf delivery.

We placed the equipment carefully in position. Leslie would handle the ratchet, and I would guide the calf up and over the pelvis. It was somewhat difficult to remove the rest of this calf. Besides being bloated and large, the calf's hair was lying in the opposite direction of the pull. It was dry, too, and we had to stop often to apply lubricant. Finally, though, the carcass popped free of the cow. A large volume of foul, bloody liquid flowed from the cow, followed by fragments and sections of the rotting afterbirth. The calf delivery looked like a success, in light of the circumstances.

Mr. Duvall pounded his cane hard onto the ground behind me. "You did it!" he exclaimed. "You got it out of her without a C-section!"

Virtie clapped her hands together once and grinned happily at me. I stood up—tired, filthy, smelling like the dead calf—and grinned back.

"Now we have to clean up the cow and see if she can stand up," I said. Leslie had dragged the calf puller and the remains of the calf to one side and detached the chains. I went to help her haul the equipment to the pickup, where we would clean it up before stowing it in the bed.

The cow was actually looking brighter. She belched loudly and cast her eyes back toward the humans behind her. She wrinkled her nose at the smell of her calf, extending her neck toward it. She snuffled. Satisfied that the calf was dead, she settled back and made no attempt to stand up.

Leslie and I gathered the supplies we'd need to flush the cow's uterus of the disintegrating placenta and the antibiotic uterine boluses that would be placed in the womb, as well as an injection of antibiotic and a calcium/magnesium IV to speed her recovery from the ordeal. We did our work quickly and efficiently and then stepped back from the cow. The moment of truth had come.

I shushed at the cow, flapping my hand towel at her head, encouraging her to stand. She ignored me.

"Use this," Mr. Duvall suggested, passing the long cattle prod to me. I took it, and before applying it anywhere on the cow, I tested it for power. It buzzed menacingly. The cow heard it and was motivated immediately to action. She sucked in a quick breath and lunged forward, hoping to escape the sting of the hot shot. I didn't even need to touch her with it.

She didn't gain her feet on that first attempt, but she gave it a powerful try. She got almost up, but the weakness in her rear end from two days of a calf pressing on her pelvic nerves and two days of labor prevented her from standing up all the way. She sank back to her chest, her eyes now full of worry over the cattle prod that had buzzed the warning to her. I set the appliance to one side.

"She'll be able to get up in awhile," I told the Duvalls. "Let her rest. She's had a hard two days." Leslie and I retired to the truck to clean the calving equipment and put it away.

The cow did stand up, but it took her three days to recover enough to do so. The Duvalls diligently brought her water and food during that time, urging her to get up, so the circulation in her legs would not be compromised. She was wobbly for a long time afterward but did remain on the Diamond D Ranch. Within six months, she conceived again. Her second calf was born normal and healthy nine months later.

I saw that cow almost every time I returned to the Duvalls, but only as she grazed in the pasture with her herd mates. She never had another experience like her first calving and was a good, productive cow for years afterward.

❖

The Duvalls were delighted with my work that day. Over the ensuing years I did many other veterinary jobs for them, all of them successful. As a matter of fact, I considered them my "charmed" ranch—everything I did for them, regardless of how ominous the call sounded, turned out well.

I decided it was that long drive to their place that did it. It allowed me a lot of time to pray for help and to consider treatment options for the case I would be tending. I had time to forget the worries of the clinic and concentrate on what I would be doing next. And it allowed time for a gathering of the forces whose job it was to keep me safe and assist me in my work.

A Grandmother and
Her Grandson

God made all the creatures and gave them our love and our fear,
To give sign, we and they are His children, one family here.
—Robert Browning

Once in practice for myself, I answered just about any call for help that I could. I tried to treat the people and the animals equally, regardless of the owner's financial situation or the pedigree tacked on the animal. Many of my cattle clients had only small herds of cattle. Often they were retired folks trying their hands at the long-held dream of being ranchers. Those people tended to know little about cows and made for interesting work.

My favorites, though, were the older folks who had lived their entire lives on family homesteads and kept a few head of cattle for extra income or for milk and meat. Some of the most interesting calls I went out on came from elderly country folks seeking help with their animals.

❖

One afternoon I took a phone call from a Ruthie Washington. With the trembling voice of an old woman, she told me she had a cow needing help; it was having trouble "finding" its calf. I was a

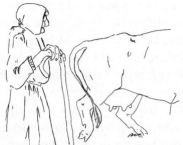

little confused as to why the lady was calling me about a lost calf and asked her to explain.

"She's been trying to find her calf since this morning," Mrs. Washington repeated. "She's been trying real hard, too. I need someone to come help her. It's her first calf."

While I continued to puzzle over why a veterinarian might be needed to help find a missing calf, Mrs. Washington added another clue to her message.

"There's one little foot showing," she said softly. "All that pushing and that's all that cow can find."

Ah! I suddenly understood what the lady was telling me. Her cow was in labor and had not been able to produce the calf. One foot was all that showed for all the cow's efforts, and the owner was worried. "Finding her calf" was evidently a quaint expression the more respectful older people used to refer to a cow in labor.

Mrs. Washington had a right to be worried; cows as well as their calves can die from a difficult delivery. I agreed to come to her assistance and asked if the cow was penned. Mrs. Washington assured me that the cow was caught up in a lot. She had a grandson, too, who would be there soon to lend assistance.

She gave me directions to her place in a breathy voice that sounded like it was the most use she'd given her vocal cords in a while. By the time she finished describing the twists and turns of the various roads I would be traveling, she sounded exhausted. I was happy she had a grandson to help out. I checked my pickup for the supplies I would need, and headed out into the country.

Ruthie Washington was just as old as her voice suggested, if not older. She was waiting patiently on her front porch when I pulled up, a frail-looking black woman with thin white hair. She was wearing a mid-calf lightweight cotton frock and a worn sunbonnet, common enough attire for the elderly farm women I worked for over the years in Houston County.

She stood up cautiously, using a walking cane made from a gnarled oak branch to help her. We introduced ourselves, and she expressed her gratitude for my willingness to help her.

"Call me Miz Ruthie," she suggested. Her grandson had not arrived to help yet, and she was apologetic and agitated about that.

"Where's the cow?" I asked, thinking if it were in the pen, I could get to work with or without the grandson to help.

"She's in the lot behind the house," Miz Ruthie said, waving with her cane in the general direction. "We can go on down there."

"I'd like to see the cow," I said, "so I know what I'll need to get from my truck to help her."

Miz Ruthie nodded in understanding and started down the steps carefully. She didn't talk much, putting her strength into making the slow trek to the barn behind the house. I walked beside her, on guard to offer a supporting hand if she needed it.

I had a special place in my heart for elderly country folk, who tried hard to hold on to their independence, their way of life, and their little plots of land. Often, with no one to help them, their facilities fell into disrepair. I never knew what I was going to find on these backwoods establishments. More often than not, the pens were in poor condition with weak fencing and what seemed like just pure luck keeping the animal confined. Sometimes I got a surprise, with a well-maintained pen as my workspace, but that was not the case this time.

The pen Miz Ruthie promised the cow would be in was not exactly a pen. It was more a small pasture at least four acres in size, surrounded by ratty, rusting barbwire. The heifer, a smallish Hereford-crossbred type, was pacing the fence, worrying after her herd mates that were out of sight in the real pasture.

The cow had a distinct wobble in her stride, no doubt from the pressure of the calf on her pelvic nerves. This I considered a factor in my favor. Veterinary school had not taught me how to throw a rope, and no amount of desire would make a cowhand out of a lariat-challenged person. Anything that would slow a cow down and make a rope catch more likely was a good thing.

There was a lean-to shed in one corner of the pasture, enclosed by an interesting-looking fence. On closer inspection, the fence was revealed to be old, rusty bedsprings, stripped of their fabric and padding and tied end-to-end with baling wire to form a barrier of sorts. I had my doubts the fence could hold the cow, especially when there was a stranger in green coveralls chasing her while wildly slinging a rope. I wondered where that grandson was.

As if reading my thoughts, Miz Ruthie glanced back toward the house and said, "Michael should be along any time now."

We both turned and looked toward the house hopefully. No one was there, no sound of an engine drifted up the road to the house. We studied the road silently, willing the young man to appear. I sighed.

"Miz Ruthie, I'm going to bring my truck around and park it near that lean-to," I said. "Then I'll see if I can't walk that cow up to the pen."

She nodded and began to slow-step her way toward the shade of the shed. I hurried back toward my pickup and got in. Before cranking the engine, I hopefully searched the road for the grandson. No telltale motor hum, no cloud of dust announcing his imminent arrival. I fired up the truck, put it in gear, and trundled it over to the pen.

When I cut off the rumbling diesel engine, I could hear a soft crooning drifting over the pasture. Miz Ruthie stood by the gate leading into the bed-spring pen, holding a feed bucket with one hand while supporting herself with the cane in her other hand. She was calling to the heifer, who stood facing the lean-to, ears pitched forward toward Miz Ruthie. I sat in my truck, waiting to see if the little cow would respond by going to her mistress. I watched as the cow's backend swayed gently from side to side. She humped up and strained against the calf. When the contraction ended, she lowed to Miz Ruthie and began to waddle across the pasture toward the pen. I stayed where I was, careful not to do anything that might cause the cow to bolt away from the lean-to. Miz Ruthie continued to coo softly to the approaching cow.

Behind me, I heard the sound of an engine and turned to see a small-sized pickup flying up the dirt road to the house, a huge cloud of red dust hanging in the air behind it. What bad timing, I thought. Just as the cow gets to the pen, here comes someone to scare her away.

Luckily, I was wrong. Apparently the pickup was a known quantity to the heifer. She did not slow her swaying pace toward the pen and, in a minute, had slid through the gate and accepted a range cube, a type of cattle feed, from the bucket Miz Ruthie held. A handsome young black man emerged from the newly arrived pickup. He was dressed in a clean T-shirt bearing the logo for a local gym, blue jeans, and high-topped sports sneakers, with a black do-rag tightened down over his close-cropped hair.

This must be Michael, I thought. He stood, unsmiling, for a moment and assessed the situation before him. He solemnly nodded to me and then hustled toward the old woman in the pen. He quietly and quickly slid behind the cow and blocked the opening back into the pasture with one of the old bedsprings leaning against the fence. The cow was now in a pen about thirty feet square with the small lean-to in one corner.

I got out of my truck. Instantly, the heifer jerked her head up and stopped chewing, eyeing me suspiciously. She turned away, heading for the now-closed gap in the bedspring fence. The moment of truth. Would she attempt to jump or push her way out? She did not. She stopped, blew loudly out her nose, and shook her head. Miz Ruthie had started her slow, stately walk back toward the gate that opened into her backyard. The young man hurried across the lot, meeting us at the gate.

"This here's Michael, my grandson," Miz Ruthie informed me. "Michael helps me with the cows sometimes. He ain't never been here for a birthin'. Michael, you got to help the doctor. Do like she tells you, mind you."

"Yes, Gramma," Michael replied, nodding respectfully. He and I looked each other up and down, wondering which of us was going to help the other.

"We need to catch the cow," I said to Michael. "Can you rope?"

Michael pursed his lips, looked down, and made a mark in the dust with the toe of his sneaker.

"No, ma'am," he answered. "Never could."

"Me neither," I acknowledged sadly. "But let's see what we can do."

I passed my rope from my left hand to my right. Even though I am left-handed, most ropes, because of the way the fibers are twisted in the construction of the rope, are made to be thrown right-handed. I figured that was part of the reason I was a poor roper. I didn't have a left-handed rope, so I had to throw right-handed. I was not very good at it. Nonetheless, some days I got lucky, and the rope went where I wanted it to.

That day was such a day. The heifer, concentrating on a contraction, was standing humped up and motionless, her tail half-raised, her eyes unfocused, and her jaws stopped mid-chew. She wasn't that far away. I had a chance of catching her. I shook out a length of the rope, gripped it firmly, gave it a half-twirl over my head, and sent it sailing toward the cow. It settled over her horns neatly. Almost in surprise, I jerked the slack and tightened the rope snuggly. I had caught the cow and made it look like I knew what I was doing. If Miz Ruthie or Michael were surprised or impressed, they didn't show it.

The next trick was to find a post stout enough to secure the rope to. The cow was actually cooperating nicely, as if she knew that help was on the way. One of the lean-to's support posts appeared to be the most suitable. I moved toward the cow's hip, shushing at her to move her toward the post. She did so quietly, allowing me time to wrap a loop of the rope around the post. With the rope snugged down around her horns, a halter around her head would not be necessary. She stood quietly as a contraction held her attention. I scooted out of the pen to my truck for supplies.

Michael followed me over and helped carry the equipment. His eyes got a little big as I assembled the calf puller I figured I'd be using. I put the chains in a bucket. Michael gulped slowly. I got the OB sleeves and lube, and we carried it all into the pen.

My first tentative exploration of the cow's inner pelvis, though gentle, was enough to cause her to fall, stiff-legged, over on her side and begin to strain fiercely against the pressure. Michael jumped to one side, alarmed. He had looked stunned when I worked my gloved arms into the cow, searching for the reason the calf could not emerge from its mother. When the cow fell over, it probably looked like I had killed her. It was obvious he had never witnessed an assisted calving.

"She all right?" Miz Ruthie called to me.

"Yes, ma'am," I answered. "She's in pretty heavy labor, though."

The calf's head was right there, positioned between its knees in the pelvic canal. I put two fingers into the calf's mouth and got a strong suckle reflex in return.

"The calf's alive," I reported. "We're going to try to get him out now."

The calf was in the proper position, just a little tight and a wee bit large. I felt confident that with a little help, the calf could be delivered in short order. I had Michael pass me a chain, which I affixed to one foreleg. After freeing up the other front leg, I asked for another chain, which Michael passed over to me quickly. I ran one hand up behind the head of the calf; it felt right. Now for the delivery.

I attached a handle to each of the chains and gave them to Michael. He looked at them speechlessly.

"When I say pull, pull whichever chain I say, left or right," I instructed. "Pull steady, no jerking. Okay?"

"Okay," Michael nodded. With his eyes wide and his long fingers closing tightly over the handles, he eased back into a brace, ready to pull.

The heifer moaned and twisted around when traction was applied to the chains, straining to deliver the calf. After a moment's hesitation, the calf's forelegs emerged, one slightly in front of the other. Just the tip of its nose emerged also. The nostrils twitched. That was as far as it got, with Michael leaning back and pulling for all he was worth. I joined him, but the calf didn't budge. It was time to get the mechanical calf puller.

I sent Michael over to get the puller from where it leaned against the fence. He was puzzled about it and watched silently as I placed it in the proper position against the cow's butt. I hooked up the chains and indicated to Michael to step up.

"I'm going to guide the calf's head out," I told him. "I want you to work the lever on this puller when I say and stop when I say, all right?" He nodded gravely.

With the cow lying on the ground as she was, I had to kneel down behind her to work. I passed my right hand into the cow and cupped my fingers behind the calf's ears. With my say-so, Michael began a slow ratcheting of the puller, coupled with a downward push on the long bar. With the extra traction, the calf's body began to slide out easily. With my hand behind it, the head came free. The calf's eyes sprang open, his mouth opened, and a lusty bawl sounded. A second later, the entire calf was on the ground, wiggling and wet. The cow heaved, and a gush of fluid flooded from her. She sat up when the calf bawled a second time, answering it with a bawl of her own.

I dragged the newborn calf a little way away from the cow, removed the chains from its legs, and helped it sit up on its chest. The cow stayed where she was, resting. I cleaned up the calf's nose, satisfied with the outcome of the procedure. With Michael's help, I hauled my equipment back to the truck. We returned to the pen, where Miz Ruthie stood watching the cow and calf from outside the salvaged bedspring fence.

I went to the cow and removed the rope from her horns. After a moment, she heaved to her feet, swayed, and then went to her calf. I joined Miz Ruthie and Michael, and we watched the cow snuffle over her calf as it attempted to rise to its feet.

"Well, grandson," Miz Ruthie said to the young man standing next to her, her hands crossed and resting on the top of her cane. "What do you think of that?"

The youth shook his head solemnly.

"I know if I was that cow," he stated, "I'd stay as far away from a bull as I could from here on."

The old woman stamped the ground fiercely with her cane, twisted around to face her grandson, and looked him in the eye. She poked him firmly in the center of his chest with a bony finger.

Nose to nose with him, from between clenched teeth, she hissed, "And you *remember* that, next time you go take a young girl out on a date!"

The work was interesting, but the people made it memorable.

Another Grandmother and Her Four Grandsons

> *I could not have slept tonight if I'd left that helpless creature to perish.*
> —Abraham Lincoln, in response to friends who chided him for delaying them when he stopped to pick up a fallen bird.

Actually, many of my clients were elderly. A number of them had been born and raised in Houston County, a few right there on the very land they ranched. The cows they fed were usually only few in number. The cows often had pet names and were spoken of fondly by their owners. I'm sure the lives these people lived, going out daily to tend to the needs of their small herds, contributed to their longevity. Over the years I was to meet and work for many senior citizens living full lives on small farms and ranches across the county. They were, truly, my favorite type of client. They were almost all honest, hardworking individuals who expected nothing less from others. Their sense of decency was strong, as well as their pride in their independence.

❖

I broke my left foot in the late spring of 1991. The four bones in the instep were crushed by one of my own horses in a freaky inci-

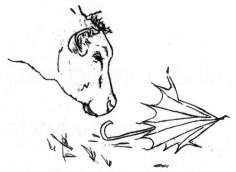

dent. It wasn't the horse's fault, and it might not even have been my fault. At any rate, I ended up with a cast on my leg that reached from my toes to my knee.

While it was inconvenient to be crippled while practicing small-animal medicine, doing large-animal work while sporting a twenty-pound plaster cast made things really difficult. The cast was heavy and itchy. It was bad enough having to wear it when I hobbled down to the barn to take care of my own horses and other animals, but I couldn't picture myself clunking around in the cast in field conditions, doing cattle or horse work for others. I decided to forego my large-animal work, in the field or at the clinic, until the cast was removed in eight weeks.

Most of my cattle and horse clients were very understanding. Those needing routine care for their animals were willing to wait until my bones had mended. Emergency calls were referred to one of the other veterinary clinics in town.

Much as I regretted having to refer my clients elsewhere for their emergency needs, I must admit I was not unhappy about it personally. It was summer, after all. While winter weather can make field work miserable, the heat of the Texas summers made it pure hell. Temperatures in the 100-degree range were not uncommon even in early June. The humidity often increased the heat index to nearly unbearable heights. Add in the heat's accentuation of smells, the hoards of flies and mosquitoes at the height of their breeding season, and no, I wasn't missing the field calls that summer much at all.

I'd made it to early July, the cast encasing my leg for seven weeks. One more week and I'd be free of that plaster torture device. One more week and I could throw away the coat-hanger wire I used to get at the itches. One more week and I could wash the sweat and accumulated dead skin cells from my leg. One more week and I could shave my leg again. Ah.

And then, just before the Fourth of July, my receptionist, Leslie, took a call from an elderly woman. Her name was Hattie McCloud, and she had never used our services before. She had a cow in labor that needed help. Leslie explained the situation with my cast and suggested the woman call one of the other veterinarians in town. She gave her their phone numbers.

A few minutes later, the phone rang again. It was Hattie McCloud. She had called all the other veterinarians, she said, but not one of them was available to help her. As a matter of fact, she'd been told that all the other veterinarians were out of town for the holiday. She wanted to know if there was any way I could help her.

Leslie handed me the phone. She thought that I might be able to convince the woman of the hindrance my injury was to my work, since she'd been unable to get the message across.

"Mrs. McCloud?" I inquired, while running the hanger wire down the inside of my cast. "Did you understand what Leslie told you? Did she tell you why I can't come out to help you?"

"Yes, she did," responded Mrs. McCloud, in a soft, gentle voice. "And I understand about your broken foot. But I need some help out here with my cow. I have four grandsons to help you, if you'll only come. If you tell one of them what to do, maybe he can help my cow."

I shook my head at Leslie, who was watching me out of the corner of her eye.

"Mrs. McCloud, that probably won't work. A trained veterinarian or someone else with experience needs to be there to pull that calf. There's no one to help you?"

"No one," Mrs. McCloud replied in a mournful whisper. "This is a good cow. She'll die if she don't get that calf out. I'm sure my grandsons can help. They are good boys, nice and strong, too. They's already here. Could you please come on out?"

I was a sucker for a sob story in those days. Still am, I guess. I didn't know what to say to this desperate lady. I couldn't think of anyone I knew who might be able to help her out. I chewed on my lower lip, wondering what to do.

"Doctor?" came the smoky old voice. "Will you come?"

I stood up.

"Give me directions out to your place, Mrs. McCloud," I said. "And make sure that cow is in a pen or has a rope on her before I get there."

The gratitude was evident in the woman's voice as she gave me precise directions to her farm. I wrote them down, told her I'd be there as soon as possible, and hung up the phone.

"I can't believe you're going out there," Leslie stated, shaking her head.

"Well, what else can I do?" I asked. "No one else is around to go. I can't let the cow die."

"What about your cast?" Leslie asked, hands on hips.

"I'll take some plastic bags and wrap it up so it won't get dirty," I answered.

"Well, don't get stepped on again," she replied grimly, as I hobbled away to prepare for the run to the country.

It was close to noon and hot outside. The blast of humid air as I stepped out the door of the clinic nearly sent me reeling. What the heck was I thinking? I checked the contents of my truck and then went back in the clinic to change into my cow clothes.

Normally for call-outs, I wore a coverall—one of those short-sleeved jumpsuits that covered a person neck to ankle—over my jeans and a T-shirt. I knew the work ahead would be grueling in this steamy hot weather. I hoped the cow was tied under a nice, big shade tree. I hoped Mrs. McCloud had a pitcher of iced tea at the ready. I hoped the calf was situated so that a flick of my wrist would straighten the bad position, and I would be out of there—

clean, dry, and my cast intact. I always hoped for the best in an unknown situation.

I tend to develop heat-stress symptoms rather easily when the heat index is high, as it was that day. I decided to wear just the coverall with no jeans or T-shirt underneath, to try to keep a little cooler. I put on an old sneaker on my right foot and was ready to go.

Hattie McCloud lived in a little family community about ten miles out of town. She was obviously the matriarch of the extended family who lived in a collection of mobile homes and small frame houses on the farm. The land had been homesteaded probably a century earlier. There were a number of such communities in Houston County. I liked going out to them. There was something enviable about having members of your family— brothers, sisters, cousins, aunts, and uncles—living nearby to help out in your daily life.

I found the row of mailboxes that marked the entrance to the McCloud property. A young black man waited in the shade of a large pecan tree near the gate. He quickly opened the gate when he understood I was the one he waited for. He indicated a house just up the lane as my destination.

Mrs. McCloud's home was a rambling old house in need of paint and a couple of braces under the roof of the front porch. A small flower plot in the front yard bloomed with a profusion of colors, obviously tenderly weeded and watered through the summer heat. Mrs. McCloud was seated in a metal yard chair on the shady front porch. She stood up as I braked in the driveway.

Mrs. McCloud was a black woman, who looked to be at least ninety years old. She was tiny and bent from age and the trials of her life. She wore a thin cotton dress that reached to mid-calf. An old-fashioned sunbonnet shielded her thinly haired head from the heat of the sun. Looking out of place on the old woman in her dated clothing was a pair of brand new, sparkling white running shoes, laced over crew socks that went halfway up the lady's thin old legs. Moving carefully, leaning on her cane and the banister to the porch, she came down the steps to greet me.

The young man who had opened the gate for me strode up. From inside the house came another young black man, tall and serious-looking.

"Mrs. McCloud, I'm Dr. Cooper-Chase," I introduced myself after I had hobbled around to the front of the truck. She nodded, barely touching my extended hand.

"Hattie," she said. "Folks call me Miz Hattie. These are my grandsons, Will and John. They'll take you down to the cow."

She looked down at my cast-enclosed leg. "I am so sorry about your injury, and I can't thank you enough for coming out here," she said, ever so softly. "No one else would come."

"I'm glad I could," I replied sincerely. "I'll come back to you here on the porch when we're finished with the cow and let you know what we found."

Not one to expend energy unnecessarily talking on a hot Texas day, Miz Hattie nodded. She indicated with her cane to the young men to go with me. Will, the taller of the two men, stepped up to me.

"The cow's in the pasture behind the house," he informed me. "We got a rope on her, but she can't get up. Just follow me around in your truck."

"Do you want a ride?" I asked them.

"No, ma'am," they both answered in unison.

"It ain't far," John said. "We'll walk." They turned and started around the house in long strides. I got back in the truck to follow.

Just behind the house was a small field. Will held the gate open for me. About fifty yards inside the fence lay a large, dairy-type cow, propped up on her chest. She was in obvious distress. Between her attempts to deliver her calf and the heat, she was showing signs of exhaustion. She panted, open-mouthed, stopping when necessary to grunt against a contraction.

Two more young black men, teenagers, stood beside her. They had thoughtfully provided the cow with a bucket of water and a small flake of hay, for which she had no interest in her present condition.

And, unfortunately, she was lying out in the direct noonday sun. The nearest shade tree was at least fifty feet away.

I stopped my pickup within fifteen feet of the cow. She paid me no heed. I got out and made a quick assessment of her overall condition. The grass in the field was short, dry, and brittle, and it crackled as I humped my cast-enclosed leg over it. The ground was hard and dry. It radiated the sun's heat back, and the air shimmered with the humidity. Sweat was gleaming on the brows of all the young men, and their shirts were beginning to dampen. I could already feel rivulets of perspiration running down my sides inside the coverall. I wiped my brow and upper lip free of sweat. A heat-induced headache was sure to develop before long, I knew. I had to get to work.

With assistance from John, I got my water jugs, soap, and gloves from my truck. I carefully positioned my wounded leg as I knelt behind the cow. After a quick vaginal examination of the cow, I stood up again. The calf was presented with its front legs folded at the knees. I'd have to correct their position before the cow could deliver. I hobbled back to my truck for the chains and handles, explaining to the young men what my intentions were.

First, though, I took a plastic trash bag and a roll of duct tape I'd brought along for the purpose and wrapped my cast protectively in the bag, taping it firmly in place. I pulled my bandanna out of my hip pocket and tied it over my head.

They were a quiet grouping of young men. Serious, unsmiling faces listened to me explain what I wanted each of them to do. Once I had corrected the position of the calf's legs, I would place a chain on each leg. John and Will would each have an OB handle to attach to a chain. Theodore, one of the teenagers, would stand at the ready with the OB lube, to replenish the supply to my gloved hands. Darius, the other teenager, would stay by the cow's head, directing her should she try to rise and leave. Each nodded solemnly in understanding.

I sure wished we were under one of those tall, shady trees. I looked wistfully over at one, the leaves fluttering in the gentle breeze passing through. I took a deep breath and knelt down, gloved, behind the cow.

It was hot work. The calf was alive and resisted my intervention in her life. Twice I'd have a small hoof in my hand and would be working it carefully up over the pelvis when the calf would wrest it away. When I finally got one foot in the proper position and attached to a chain, the cow strained mightily, causing the calf's head to emerge from the uterus and into the birth canal. Still, with one bent leg, the calf wasn't going to be able to come out. I had to hold the calf back each time the cow strained to prevent it from being wedged more tightly in the birth canal, and then go back to work trying to position the other leg.

Sweat was pouring off me. I couldn't see for the salty fluid flowing into my eyes. I couldn't wipe my eyes, either, not with messy plastic gloves on my hands and arms. Flies, attracted by the cow's blood and vaginal fluid, buzzed around and landed on my face. I could not swipe at them. I had to keep working.

At one point, my good leg braced against the ground as I pushed to hold the calf against the straining cow, I glanced around me. Each of the young men was waiting to help, silent, tensed, so solemn in appearance I almost chuckled. Behind us, coming from the house through the small back yard, was Miz Hattie. She carried a red-and-white striped umbrella over her head, while steadying herself with her cane. Her gleaming white sneakers flashed in the sun. She carefully opened the gate, crossed into the field, shut the gate, and turned to move cautiously toward us.

I was still lying on the ground behind the cow, working to free the calf's other leg, while I watched the old lady walking carefully across the field, that bright umbrella shading her, those shoes reflecting the sun's rays into my eyes. The calf's foot moved just enough, and it suddenly slid into position. I got it; I drew it out into the light of day and quickly looped a chain over the fetlock, handing the other end to Will.

"Okay," I said to Will and John, who held the OB handles, now attached to the chains, "when I say, pull slow and steady. Don't jerk on the chain, just pull slow and steady unless I say otherwise." Each young man nodded in understanding.

I put one hand back into the cow and found the calf's chin. I guided it to sit between the front legs.

"Slow and easy," I instructed.

Slowly, carefully, they pulled on the calf, first John, then Will, as I indicated. The calf's nose popped into the hot air and the nostrils wrinkled. The cow gave a heave, and the calf slid out, easily, onto the ground. Will and John dragged the calf, a light-brown heifer, a few feet from the cow.

The young men began to smile, laugh with relief, and slap each other on the back, all the while admiring the calf. I cautioned Darius not to leave his post by the cow's head, as now was the time she would be most inclined to get up. But the cow ignored her calf and made no attempt to get up. She merely panted in the heat.

By this time, Miz Hattie had made her slow way over to where her grandsons were removing the OB chains from the calf. She held her umbrella out to shade the calf from the sun's intense rays.

I stood up. My plaster-encased leg felt like it weighed a hundred pounds. Moisture had fogged the plastic bag and sweat had puddled inside it. I tore at the tape to remove the bag. The plaster cast felt soggy from the soaking it had gotten from my perspiration. My coveralls were drenched in sweat. I was drenched, too, my scalp prickling from the heat. Wow. The heat-induced headache that had knocked at the back of my eyes earlier was now kicking in the door.

Miz Hattie was smiling slightly, nudging the wiggling calf with her cane. The four young men were standing in a semicircle, laughing lightly and exclaiming at the sight, pleased to have participated in the event. I wondered if any of them realized I was still there.

I tiredly bent to pick up a chain and take it to the truck. I got some medicine for the cow and hobbled over to give her an injection in the neck. She bawled low and attempted to get up. I backed away to give her the room she needed. Awkwardly, the cow staggered up on all fours, trailing the pink membrane of afterbirth behind her. She did not seek her calf, but merely stood, head extended, panting in the heat.

"Put the calf where she can see it," I suggested, coming around to stand next to Miz Hattie. The two teenagers hefted the calf and carried it carefully to the front of the cow.

The cow suddenly stopped her panting and snuffled in the direction of the calf. A look of comprehension came to her eyes, and she emitted a low hum, a gentle, quiet sound I loved to hear a mama cow sing. She reached out with her long tongue and tasted the little heifer. She began to sing in earnest, washing the calf tenderly with long swipes of her rough tongue. It was pretty to see.

❖

My headache receded a little bit. I stood there watching the cow and calf with Miz Hattie, her four grandsons strung out in a line beside her.

Suddenly, unexpectedly, and with a lot more energy than I expected from an ancient woman, Hattie McCloud screeched piercingly. She raised her arms and began to beat her grandsons with her umbrella in one hand and her cane in the other. I was speechless, aghast, watching her flail at those four young men. They were jumping back from her, looks of utter confusion on their faces. They put their arms up to shield their heads from her onslaught, voices raised in objection.

"No, Gramma!"

"What did I do?"

"Ow, ow!"

What the hell was going on? Her screeching began to sound like words to me. I made out, "Don't you look at her! Don't you look at that woman!"

What? What the heck was she telling them? They hadn't been looking at me; they had been watching the cow and calf! I looked down at myself, wondering what it was she didn't want them to see.

I was soaking wet. My coveralls, a light gray when dry, were soaked and dark with sweat and were plastered to me everywhere except in two places. Dry outlines of my bra and panties stood out in light-gray relief where my underwear had prevented the coveralls from getting soaked.

I quickly plucked at the coveralls, releasing the fabric from my skin, shaking them loose. Miz Hattie had stopped assailing her grandsons and was huffing and blowing for breath.

"Miz Hattie, it's all right," I assured her, attempted to mollify her by gently patting her bony shoulder. "They didn't see anything. They didn't even look at me. They didn't do anything wrong."

The old lady patted her brow with a handkerchief she had produced from one sleeve. She glared menacingly at her grandsons as she leaned on her cane. Her umbrella lay half-open and broken on the ground. The four young men had retreated beyond her reach, trying to make themselves look small. Each was making a concentrated effort not to look in my direction.

"I ain't gonna have no grandchild of mine gettin' in trouble for looking at a white woman's underwear," Miz Hattie declared. She looked me up and down. "You come out here again, young lady, you best wear some clothes under that suit."

"Yes, ma'am," I said, chastised. I continued to pull the wet fabric away from my skin, trying to make it look baggy, as I went to pick up my equipment.

"Let these young men do dat," Miz Hattie said to me. She barked at her grandsons. "Git over here and help this lady with this stuff!"

All four of them jumped at her instructions and, keeping a wide berth of their grandmother, circled around to pick up what little equipment had been left on the ground.

"And don't none of you look at her!" she snapped, waving her cane. Each ducked his head and averted his eyes as they scurried around.

"Now," Miz Hattie drew herself up as straight as she could. The top of her bonneted head barely reached my shoulder. "How much do I owe you for your work?"

I quoted her a price, and she sent her youngest grandson to the house for her change purse. He galloped off quickly. The other three were at a loss as to what to do. They waited nervously, eyes down, occasionally throwing a glance at their grandmother. I was embarrassed for them as well as myself.

Darius came loping back with his grandmother's purse. She carefully counted out the bills and gave me my wages. She signaled to Theodore, who scurried to stand in front of her, awaiting orders.

"Open the gate for this woman," she told him. She waved her cane at the others, causing them to duck defensively. "You all git that cow and calf in some shade and get her some water and some range cubes to eat."

The four grandsons scattered like leaves before a gale-force wind to do their grandmother's bidding.

She turned back to me. Her face, a moment ago tight and angry, was relaxed and smiling gently.

"Thank you for coming," she said, her voice once again soft and lilting, although a little bit raw from shouting. "I won't forget your kindness."

❖

I knew I wouldn't forget the incident either. I realized as I pulled out of the gate, waving to Theodore as I left, that I no longer had a pounding headache. I drove back to the clinic, cheered and satisfied that I'd done the right thing by responding to Mrs. McCloud's desperate plea for help with her cow.

I also vowed I would, from that day forward, always wear shorts and a shirt under my coveralls on call-outs on hot, humid summer days.

Part 4

All in a

Day's Work

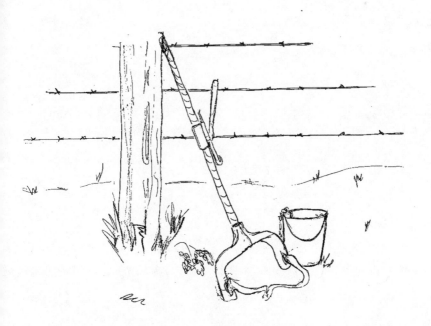

Mr. Allbright's Choking Cow

When a man has pity on all living creatures then only is he noble.
　　　　　　　　　　　　　　　　　　　—Buddha

I don't wear a wedding ring, for the simple reason I lost it one night during a calf delivery. Usually I would remove it, hang it from a hook on the turn-signal lever in the truck, and replace it on my finger once I crawled back into the cab for the return home. That fateful evening, however, I'd forgotten to take it off, and during the indelicate work of extracting the slippery calf from the cow, the ring, well lubricated by the amniotic fluid and my obstetric lube, slid from my finger and vanished into the soil and debris of the ranch lot. It was never recovered and I never replaced it. So, wedding-ring-less, many people who didn't know me or my husband didn't realize I had a spouse keeping the home fires burning while I was out on a job.

❖

One night, close to midnight, while we were hard asleep in our bed, the phone rang. Jack awoke to the jangle first. Since the telephone rested on the table next to his side of the bed, he reached out, fumbled a bit, picked up the receiver, and muttered a groggy "Hello?" Also jogged from a very sound sleep, I lay still, eyes closed, praying it was a wrong number.

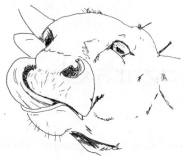

After a quiet pause of several seconds, Jack repeated his "Hello?" After another wait, he hung up.

"Wrong number, I guess," he informed me. "Whoever it was didn't say a thing."

Fine with me. I snuggled deeper in the covers. I really didn't want to go out to see a sick or injured animal. I just wanted to sleep.

It was not to be. A couple of minutes later the phone shrilled again, seemingly louder without the muffle of dreams between it and my ears. Jack, jarred awake again, picked up the receiver.

"Hello," he stated, this time just a little peeved. A pause. "Yes, she's here," he replied to an inquiry. I moaned.

"Who is it?" I asked.

"A Mr. Allbright," Jack said. "He asked if Dr. Cooper-Chase was here."

I took the phone, and grunted a cheerless greeting into it.

"Dr. Cooper-Chase?" a man asked cautiously.

"Yes," I confirmed his suspicions.

"Frank Allbright here," he said. "I hate to disturb you when you, uh, have company, but I have a cow in trouble."

Company? I sat up and turned on the bedside lamp. What did he mean by company? I glanced over at Jack, who lay on his back, shielding his eyes from the sudden rude glare of the light.

"Mr. Allbright, don't worry about it," I said. "My husband's used to late-night calls. What seems to be the problem with your cow?"

There was silence on the other end of the line.

"Mr. Allbright?"

"Your husband? You're married?" The words came to my ear with a tone of disbelief. "Oh, that's good!" Mr. Allbright gave a short, relieved chuckle. "My cow is real sick. She can't breathe. Can you come look at her? I think she'll die before morning if she doesn't get tended tonight."

I knew Mr. Allbright, having done some work for him in the past. I knew where his ranch was, the well-kept condition of his pens, and the quality of his cows. I also knew he wouldn't call at such an hour of the night unless he thought he had a serious problem. I told him I would be there as soon as possible. He said he would have his grandson out to help and some floodlights to illuminate the pens we'd be working in. I hung up the phone.

"What was that about?" Jack asked, his arm still slung over his eyes.

"Mr. Allbright thought you were a 'guest'," I said. "Now I have to go out and look at one of his cows."

"A guest?" Jack asked, sliding his arm from his eyes to look at me.

"He didn't know I was married," I explained.

"Oh!" Jack hitched himself up onto his elbows. "That was probably him who called the first time. Hung up when he heard a man's voice!"

"Yep," I agreed, pulling on my cow clothes, readying to go examine a dypsneic cow. "Want to come along?"

Jack cast a quick eye at the clock, then flopped back flat, pulling his pillow over his head.

"Nope" was his answer. I sighed. I wished I could have done the same.

❖

The ranch wasn't far away, and Mr. Allbright had the cow in the chute but not caught in the head gate. He had a teenaged boy alongside to help. We greeted each other, and if it hadn't been a black night with only a couple floodlights beaming down onto our patient, I'm sure I would have seen that Mr. Allbright's face was a shiny red from his somewhat embarrassing call to me. I wasn't going to mention it, and apparently he decided not to, either.

I climbed up on the rails to look over at the black Angus cow standing in the chute. She looked warily up at me, heaving for breath, great ropes of bubbly saliva flowing off her jaws. Her protruding tongue appeared black in the artificial light. She definitely was having trouble breathing. To me, she appeared to be choking.

"She can't breathe," Mr. Allbright said, worriedly peering through the rails at his cow. "She was fine this afternoon. I come out this evening, and she was standing in the corner and wouldn't eat. She was coughing and slobbering a bit. I thought she had a touch of pneumonia, so I penned her up, and gave her a shot of Combiotic. She kept getting worse. I got worried and come out and checked her after Jay Leno went off. She wouldn't move and was really having a hard time breathing. That's when I called you."

Jay Leno on The Tonight Show? I didn't know ranchers stayed up late enough to watch Jay Leno, I thought to myself as I climbed up on the fence. I looked around the lot. A group of fat Angus cows, their eyes glowing green in the light, lined the pen's gate, watching the goings on in the lot.

"Any of the other cows sick?" I asked. Mr. Allbright said that none of the others were having any problems.

"Do the cows come in here to graze?" was my second question.

Mr. Allbright confirmed that they did, as the water trough that stood along one fence was their only source of water while they were grazing the connecting pasture. I noted a thin tree down the fence line.

"What kind of tree is that?" I asked.

Mr. Allbright squinted in the dark, following my pointing index finger.

"A pear tree," he said. "Them small, hard canner pears. My wife likes to cook with them. She makes a mock apple pie with them and puts some up in jars." He talked fast, nervously. More information than I needed, I thought tiredly.

"I think the cow is choking on one," I said, nodding toward the distressed cow.

Mr. Allbright's jaw fell open.

"Them cows eat the pears all the time," he informed me. "I've never seen one choke before."

"You're seeing one now," I said. "Let's catch her head so I can take a look."

With some doubt as to my diagnosis, Mr. Allbright signaled his grandson to open the head gate while he went beside the cow to coax her forward. The cow, stressed from lack of oxygen, stepped slowly forward and fitted her head quietly through the head catch of the gate, as if pleading for help. I had retrieved a set of nose tongs from my truck, as well as a powerful flashlight. With the tongs applied to the cow's nasal septum, I hoisted her head, using the overhead bar of the chute as a wrapping post for the rope of the tongs. The upward angling of her head caused the cow's mouth to gape wide. She gave a strangled bawl and attempted to cough. I shined the flashlight's beam down her throat.

There, lodged firmly in the pharynx, pressing heavily against the tracheal opening, was a slobber-covered green pear. I asked Mr. Allbright to step over and look in. He nodded grimly, a mixed look of disbelief, chagrin, and relief on his face.

"Now, we have to get it out of there," I intoned gravely.

From my truck I procured a heavy metal mouth gag called a McPherson's Speculum. Designed to allow a veterinarian to safely open and work inside a horse's mouth while floating its teeth, this gag had special mouth plates that could be substituted for the horse plates, allowing it to be used on cattle. Mr. Allbright's eyes bugged as I fitted the awkward contraption on the patient. Once the gag was in place, I was able to prop the cow's jaws wide open, allowing me a measure of safety while inserting my arm deep into the her mouth.

This was one of those times when having the small arms and hands of a woman was an advantage. With the cow's tongue working feverishly to push my hand out, I slid my left hand between the plates of the gag, over her tongue, past the huge cheek teeth to the back of her mouth. My arm was up to the elbow in the cow's oral cavity before my index finger touched the firm, pebbly surface of the hard green piece of fruit. There was just enough give in the pharyngeal wall to ease my finger past the pear. I hooked my finger behind it and began easing it out. The pressure that resulted was just enough to completely occlude the respiratory tract opening, and the cow, alarmed at suddenly being unable to breathe at all, struggled and surged forward. I stayed with her, praying the head gate and nose tongs would hold her and prevent her from slamming the heavy metal gag into my head.

The cow reared up as far as she could, which wasn't far due to the restraints on her, but as she came down she exhaled hard, and the pear, loosened by my finger, blew loose from its moorings right into the palm of my hand. I extracted my arm from the cow, triumphantly displaying the offending fruit, while the cow took in great gulps of air, reveling in unrestricted breathing for the first time in hours. It wasn't long before we were able to release the cow. She gave a little hop as she trotted back to her herd mates, bellowing loudly with full lung capacity.

❖

Mr. Allbright was delighted with the outcome of the call, and so was I. With a promise from him that he would come by in the morning to pay his bill, I left the Allbright ranch to head back home to my sleeping husband, leaving Mr. Allbright and his grandson picking up pears from the lot by glaring floodlight and handheld flashlight.

Mr. Carter's Eyesight

The soul is the same in all living creatures,
although the body of each is different.
—Hippocrates

Thankfully, not that many calls came in the dead of the night, waking me from a much-needed sleep and leaving me weary the next day. A good portion of the emergency calls came during the week, during regular waking, working hours. I had a set of good working pens at the clinic, and if possible I had the owner bring the sick cow into town where I could exam her and work on her more easily.

If a cow had to stay at the clinic for further treatment over the following days, there were good clean stalls to keep her in, with a chute to help guide the cow from the stall to the squeeze chute for treatment. Many people liked the idea of leaving the animal for us to tend, over having to deal with a sick cow on the home ranch. Not surprisingly, my older clients were often the most willing to make use of that service.

❖

The Carters were one of my favorite couple-clients. Well into their eighties, they were both robust individuals with few health problems. They had lived their entire sixty-eight years of married life on one ranch, a ranch that had belonged to Mr. Carter's parents before him.

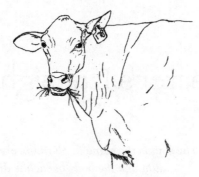

The couple maintained a half-acre vegetable garden behind their house, planted year-round in whatever the seasonal crop was. The crops grew thick and tall and so bountifully that the Carters were always giving away the produce they did not eat, can, or freeze for use later on. I was the happy recipient of many a bag of sweet corn, turnip greens, tomatoes, peppers, and other good homegrown vegetables.

They had chickens for eggs and meat, a pig to raise for slaughter, and usually a pair of turkeys for the holiday meals. I'm sure eating all that wonderful homegrown produce and livestock, plus the daily work that went into tending it all, helped account for the couple's continuing good health so far into old age.

Mrs. Carter did suffer from mild heart problems, but even at the age of eighty-five, her hearing was extremely acute and she could still read without glasses. Mr. Carter, at eighty-eight, was proud of the fact he used no prescription drugs and could read his Louis L'Amour novels with only a good light source to help him see the print on the pages.

However, he did have a hearing problem; he was profoundly deaf, actually. His hearing aids were basically useless, and you had to yell loudly for him to hear you. He could manage to hear Mrs. Carter's voice well enough, it seemed; maybe he could read her lips or maybe he was attuned to the timbre of her voice. If he came in to the clinic without her, we usually had to write notes for him to take back to his wife, to convey the findings of my examination of an animal, for medication directions, or whatever else we had to tell her, such as thank you for the bags of produce she inevitably had her husband deliver to us.

Their one son and one daughter had no interest in ranching; it was a sure thing that when the elderly Carters passed away, their herd of seventy or so cross-bred mama cows and four good Brahman bulls would be sold and the ranch land divided up and sold also. There was something sad about that, to me. All those years of work, all that dedication and love for the land and its gifts. At the end it would all be reduced to paperwork and sold in parcels. In the meantime, I could do what I could to help them keep ranching.

This particular visit to my clinic was with a large, mottled-black cow with a bad udder. She was a relatively old cow; the Carters tended to keep their cows until they died of old age. Mr. Carter would have just as soon sold the non-producers as feed them, but Mrs. Carter firmly believed that a cow that had produced a calf for them year after year deserved to live out her life on the home place. I knew they had at least one Jersey, well into her twenties, chewing cud in peace in a pasture behind the house, barren for at least the preceding five years. Bulls came and went, but the cows stayed on.

The cow presented to me this day had to be at least sixteen years old. She was fat and shiny and was nursing a rowdy bull calf. Her problem was evident as she walked calmly off the trailer, down the loading ramp, and into the holding pen behind my clinic. She was subdued and panting as if with a fever, and she had that faraway, preoccupied look suffering animals tend to get. Both of the rear quarters of her generous-sized udder were swollen, red, and painful even to look at, the teats strutted and sticking straight out to the sides. Not a pretty picture.

The cow, graced with the name of "Bonnie" by her loving lady owner, walked slowly, careful to avoid hitting the blistered-looking udder with a hind leg. After a cursory exam in the holding pen, we urged the suffering cow down the chute to the head gate.

Once the cow was secured in the iron-pipe squeeze and her head restrained by the head gate, I was able to get a better look at her condition. She had a fever of 104 degrees, no doubt a result of the infection in her udder. When she had called to schedule an appointment for the cow, Mrs. Carter had told me that Bonnie hadn't been eating well, and it looked like the calf wasn't getting much to eat. Both of these symptoms were common in lactating cows with fevers.

Though Bonnie was a gentle cow by nature and by upbringing, the tendency to kick due to pain was nonetheless there, so I applied a thick, soft rope to one of the cow's hind legs as a hobble. This simple device allowed me to exam the udder in relative safety.

While still stooped next to the cow, gently feeling over the udder, I called out to Mr. Carter.

"She's got mastitis!" No response. Mr. Carter just stood there silently, watching me work with the cow. I realized my back was to him and deduced he couldn't hear me and didn't know I was speaking to him. I stood up and turned to him.

"She's got mastitis!" I repeated to him.

Mr. Carter looked a little bewildered. He cupped his right hand over his ear to make a funnel to help take in sound.

"Huh?" he asked.

"Mastitis!" I yelled, having raised my voice an octave while pointing at the cow's angry udder. "Infected!"

Mr. Carter nodded in understanding. He'd had cows in the past with infected mammary glands. He knew what mastitis was.

"I figgered as much!" he replied, nodding. Like a lot of deaf people who could not hear even themselves, he spoke loudly. "Can we save her?"

❖

This particular cow was one of Mrs. Carter's favorites. She had bottle-fed the cow from calfhood and raised her as a pet. Even if the treatment ended up being involved and expensive, Mrs. Carter would agree to it in order to save the cow. Mr. Carter, on the other hand, did not always like treating sick animals; he might just as soon dispose of her. I figured he would have to hash that out with his wife.

"I think so," I told him. I pantomimed holding a telephone receiver to my ear. "Let me call Mrs. Carter and talk to her."

Mr. Carter understood what I was trying to say, even if he couldn't hear me. He tended to leave the decisions on what to do with the cows up to his wife. We left the cow where she was and headed into the main clinic to the phones.

I called Mrs. Carter and described my findings. As I had assumed, there was no question about treating the cow. Mrs. Carter didn't feel well herself, though, and wanted to know if I could keep the cow for a day or two and do the treatments at the clinic. At home, she'd be the one to treat the cow, as Mr. Carter didn't like that job.

"Of course," I told her. "No problem."

I would send Mr. Carter home without the cow. We'd keep the cow and treat her condition for as long as necessary. I felt certain we would see a big improvement in her udder's health within twenty-four hours, and we could send her home in two or three days. Mrs. Carter was agreeable to that.

I told Mr. Carter what I had discussed with his wife, as best I could by talking loudly and using pantomime. The message conveyed, the old man climbed into his pickup and left for home, leaving the cow, along with her calf, at the clinic for treatment.

❖

The best way to treat mastitis, besides antibiotics, is to strip all the milk from the affected quarters, if possible. Depending on the severity of the case and the cooperation of the patient, it might be an easy job, or it might not be. Bonnie proved to be very cooperative, and her condition, as bad as it looked, was not terribly severe. I was able to milk her rear quarters dry of several quarts of thick, purulent, blood-tinged milk.

With the removal of the bad milk, the relief to the cow was obvious. Since the two front quarters were not infected, the calf would be able to nurse from them. Once we got the fever down, the cow would quickly begin to produce enough milk for the calf. After removing the infected milk, I treated both the infected quarters with a medication that was injected up the teat canal into the udder. I slathered a lanolin-based udder cream onto the stretched skin of the udder to sooth it and relieve the dryness. I then used an injectable antibiotic to treat the systemic infection raging in the cow. I felt sure her fever would be down by morning and that she would be eating and producing milk.

Sure enough, the next morning Bonnie the Big, Black, Mottled Cow was bright, alert, eating heartily, and nursing her hungry calf. We walked her down the chute and into the head gate. No foot hobble was necessary to examine her udder that morning; it was more normal in color and obviously not nearly as painful. Still, I had to milk the rear quarters dry again. Blood and infection was still present in the milk, so I repeated the antibiotic treatment.

We kept the cow for a full three days, treating the udder twice a day after milking her dry. By the third day, the udder was soft and painless, the milk clean and white and infection-free. The calf was obviously getting plenty to drink, as the cow was allowing him to nurse from the rear quarters now, as well as the healthy forequarters of her udder. I decided the cow would be ready to go home after one more treatment in the evening.

I called Mrs. Carter to tell her the good news. She was overjoyed. A gentle, sweet lady, she wept a little with happiness for her cow. She promised Mr. Carter would be by the next morning with the trailer to fetch the cow and to pay the bill.

The first person to appear at the clinic the next morning was Mr. Carter with his trailer. He had carefully and expertly backed it up to the loading chute even before we knew he was there. I met him at the trailer to help him load the cow. Bonnie walked sedately and regally up the ramp into the trailer, her fat and sassy calf bucking and snorting along behind her. We shut the gate and secured the latches of the trailer.

Mr. Carter pulled a checkbook from his pocket. I pointed toward the main clinic, indicating we should go inside to the front desk where my receptionist had his bill ready. Never saying a word, he nodded in understanding, and strode into the building.

Leslie had his bill ready, and rather than yell at the old man to tell him the total, she pointed to the bill, turning it to face him so he could read the numbers himself. He studied it a moment, nodded, and wrote the check. She quickly wrote the check number on the receipt and handed it to him. He studied it a moment before folding it carefully and sliding it into his pocket.

Most of the transaction had been performed without a word being spoken. Mr. Carter was obviously not quite ready to go, though. He had a question from Mrs. Carter.

"Wilma wants to know when she can bring a cat by to be fixed," he said to me. "She told me to ask you that just before I left the house. She would have called, but she said I could ask you the question when I came for the cow."

"Okay," I said. "We can give you a date."

"What?" he asked.

I raised my voice, looking directly at him.

"We can do it on Thursday!"

He cupped his hand behind his ear.

"What?" he asked again.

I didn't want to shout any louder. I didn't figure he would be able to hear me anyway. So I picked up a note pad from the desk, along with a pen, and started to write the surgery date for the cat on the paper. Wouldn't you know, the ink gave out before I'd written two letters. I pitched the empty pen in the trash can and reached for another from the pen holder on the desk. There were no ballpoint pens in the can, however.

After pawing through the assortment of markers and pencils, I grabbed a Sharpie, a medium-point black marker, out of the pile. It was well used and the tip was blunted badly. On the paper, the letters ran into blobs unless I wrote them large. I sighed in minor frustration and wrote the note in large, blocky letters—a date, a brief set of instructions on not feeding the cat the night before the surgery, and what time to have her at the clinic. I placed the note on the counter in front of the patiently waiting Mr. Carter.

The old man picked up the note carefully, held it up, and read it top to bottom. I could see his jaw tightening, his face going a little red. What was the problem, I wondered. Was it a bad appointment date?

Suddenly Mr. Carter slammed the piece of paper down onto the counter. I jumped, Leslie jumped. Keeping his hand down hard on the paper, Mr. Carter leaned over the counter, glaring directly at me. I drew back a little. He picked the note up in his fist and shook it violently at me. I cringed.

"I'M DEAF!" he bellowed at me. "NOT BLIND!"

With that he crumbled up the note, thrust it into his shirt pocket, turned, and stomped out of the clinic.

I looked at Leslie in amazement. Obviously I had offended the old gent by writing the note in big, bold, primary-school letters. I surely had not meant to insult him.

When I saw Mr. and Mrs. Carter the following Thursday as they brought their cat in for surgery, Mr. Carter was just as friendly as he had ever been. Mrs. Carter told me that he had come home with the cow that morning very upset over that note I had written in big block letters. While she thought it was funny, he certainly had not. He was very proud of not having to wear glasses to read, she said, and that note just made him angry.

❖

I guarantee to you, I never wrote another block-letter note for Mr. Carter. I even made a point of using a fine-point pen to write any notes to him after that. You just never know what might upset an individual, that's for sure.

The Drummond Calves

Be sure you know the condition of your flocks,
give careful attention to your herds.
—Proverbs 27:23

I didn't get into veterinary medicine because I liked cows. I mean,
I *liked* cows. I liked all animals, but cows weren't my passion.
Horses were my favorite animals of all the species gifted to us
mere mortals on this earth. They still are, for that matter.

My first job as a veterinary assistant was with a clinic that did
a mixed practice. I worked with three veterinarians as they cared
for horses, cattle, dogs, and cats. That wonderful experience led
me to night classes, then to daytime college courses while I
worked at various veterinary clinics as an assistant, and eventually into the application process for veterinary school.

I was admitted into the professional curriculum at Texas A & M
College of Veterinary Medicine in the fall of 1982. It was my desire
to work with horses that drove me on and kept me focused on
gaining my degree, which I acquired in the spring of 1986. But
somehow, it was working with cows and cow people that became
one of the best parts of being a veterinarian and just about the
most fulfilling aspect of my career.

❖

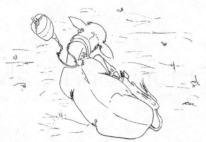

Neither rain nor hail nor sleet nor snow nor heat of day nor dark of night shall keep this carrier from the swift completion of his appointed rounds.

That quote is often attributed to the devoted industry of postal carriers, but I would wager that veterinarians who do large-animal work would argue that, in comparison to what they do for a living, postal carriers have it cushy.

While many cattle ranchers try to regulate their cattle's breeding so that calves hit the ground at the most opportune time of the year, the truth of the matter is that calves are born at any time of the year, in all kinds of weather, and in all kinds of situations. There are months when calving activity is especially high, no doubt about that, but veterinarians regularly drive out in all kinds of weather year-round to meet the challenges presented to them. Most calves are born under field conditions, with cows going into labor with no regard whatsoever for the attending veterinarian's comfort or safety.

Sick animals, too, require tending, regardless of the weather conditions. Many animals did have problems in foul weather due to the stress of cold and wet upon the old, the young, and the marginally healthy. Being a veterinarian was a responsibility as well as a job, but it had its rewards. Such was the case with the Drummonds' sick little calves.

❖

East Texas winter weather tends to be erratic. Every day is different; you just don't know what you're going to get. Snow is a rarity, but it isn't really missed by the natives. Besides, if it did snow, the snow wouldn't have a chance of staying on the ground long, if at all. The unpredictable swings between cold and warm are not at all like a northern-style winter. In this part of the state, one day might be clear and blue-skied, with low humidity and warm temperatures. The next day might be rainy and bone-chilling cold.

Often a morning begins with dark, hovering clouds and dank, cold air, but by midafternoon the temperature is summer-like, with the humidity so high you feel swimming through the air would be easier than trying to walk. It's not uncommon for homes and businesses to have both heaters and air conditioners up and running within the same twenty-four-hour period. The old saying is, "If you don't like Texas weather, just wait a minute." It's true.

On cold, rainy days, it should have been allowable to stay at home with a wood fire taking the bone-eating damp out of the air and a cup of coffee steaming on the end table, as I nestled on the sofa with the cats and a good book. At least, that's what I believed. However, for a veterinarian who practiced large-animal medicine, that wasn't always an option. When a client called, you bundled up in your insulated overalls and rubber boots, pulled on your wool cap, sucked in your gut, and walked out into the weather to make the drive to the rancher in need of assistance.

On this gloomy, late-winter morning, it was a call-out to the Drummonds' ranch, about thirty-five miles from town. I had been to the ranch many times before. The Drummonds and I had become comfortable enough with each other over the years of working together to use first names in addressing each other. While this might seem like an obvious thing—calling someone by their first name—I was born and raised in the South and brought up to address folks by their surnames as a sign of respect and deference to their age and/or life experiences.

With my elderly clients, there was usually no question about this being the thing to do. There were some elderly ladies whose given names were never revealed, as they called themselves only by their husband's name. I had one client, long dead of old age now, named Mrs. Sherman Polk. That's how she identified herself on the phone, how she signed her checks, and how she expected to be addressed, though her husband, Mr. Sherman Polk, had been dead for thirty years. One day, she handed me a check for vaccinations for her cat. It was signed "Mrs. Sherman Polk," as usual, with that name printed in the upper left corner. On impulse, I asked her what her baptized name was. She was startled. No one had ever asked her, she said. She smiled, apparently pleased that someone might show an interest in who she was. Her name was Alma.

I was well into my thirties when I opened my practice in Houston County, and many of the people who were nearer to my own age insisted that I call them by their first names, or I just did so when it seemed appropriate. There were plenty of people with whom I was never casual enough to address as anything other than Mister or Missus, regardless of their ages or what they did for a living.

I really liked the Drummonds, and happily they were friendly, informal folks, only a decade or so older than I was, who liked hearing their first names spoken, though they insisted on addressing me as Doctor or, more personally, as Doc.

Maureen and Archie had a small herd of commercial cattle with a Brahman bull as the sire. At their place, the calving problems tended to be few and uncomplicated, and this wasn't a calving call. This time it was to examine two suckling calves with profuse diarrhea.

According to Archie's call to my office, one calf appeared to be close to death, the other down and so depressed as to ignore anything done for her. The diarrhea was described to be whitish in color and foul in smell. Both calves were from first-time heifers, meaning they were the first-born calves of the mother cows. Calving had apparently been uneventful, and these two month-old calves had been thriving until this morning. Archie found the first one lying on the remnants of one of the round bales of hay he'd fed to his herd the day before. The second calf he discovered standing humped up and droopy when he returned to the field with another round bale to feed the mother cows. He had carried both calves back up to the barn lot before calling me for help. I bundled up in my warm vest and rubber boots and headed out the door.

When I got to the ranch, Maureen was at the gate to open it for me and directed me toward the barn where her husband waited nearby with the calves. I drove across the field toward the barn, the cold, misting rain keeping my truck's windshield wipers in business. Archie had both calves outside and away from the barn, on a slight hill, which appeared drier than the rest of the pasture. He had placed a plastic tarp on the ground. On this he had heaped clean, dry hay, lain the calves on the hay, heaped more hay over them in fluffy mounds for insulation, and dropped a canvas tarp over the works to protect them from the elements.

Three cows stood next to the tarp, bobbing their heads as if they were trying to peer under the tarp for a glimpse of their calves. I drove my truck up next to the tarp, cut the engine, and got out. The chilly rain beat a soft tattoo on the canvas tarp.

"I got them as dry as I could, Doc," Archie said, peeling back one corner of the tarp to show me the patients. He gestured toward the barn, set back a little down a slope. "The barn's flooded from that last big rain; nowhere dry in there. I thought this was better."

"This is fine, Arch," I said, kneeling down in the hay next to the calves. Besides the two he had told me about, I noticed a third calf lying under the tarp. It was larger, older, and in better condition than either of the first two. I looked at Arch questioningly.

"I found that little bull calf after I called you," he explained. "He's got the scours, too, but he doesn't look too bad. I almost missed seeing him. He was kinda dragging along after his mama, and when she stopped, he went to nurse her. I thought he was okay, but then he shot a stream of diarrhea out behind him six feet, I swear. You can see it all over his butt; looks just like these two. So I brought him up, too."

I nodded in understanding. The sicker of the first two calves was a little heifer, a red baldie that smelled badly of diarrhea and death. She was dehydrated and bony, probably weighing no more than eighty pounds. She was flat on her side, heaving for air, her head thrown back and her eyes rolled up so only the whites showed. A check with the digital thermometer revealed a body temperature so low it didn't register. I shook my head. The prognosis was pretty grim.

The other calf was also a heifer, but she was positioned on her chest, her head turned into her flank. A little heavier than the first and not quite as dehydrated, she appeared to be asleep and swung her head around slowly in response to my touch. Her nose was crusty and red, and the nostrils rapidly pinched closed and open again as she breathed. Her rectal temperature was a screaming 106 degrees Fahrenheit. White diarrhea, dried to a yellow hue, stained her rear and tail, while a steady stream of it leaked from her anus. The smell under the tarp was unpleasant, to say the least.

The third calf, a gray bull calf that probably weighed about 150 pounds, was bright-eyed and watchful, though it was obvious that he was also sick. He lay on his chest, head up and ears forward. He panted from a fever, and when he grunted in protest at being handled, the effort caused foul diarrhea to pour from him.

Outside the tarp, the three mother cows waited anxiously. Only the third calf's mama appeared to have been nursed recently. Her udder had a relaxed, somewhat deflated look, while the other two cows had udders strutted with milk, the skin shiny and red from the strain. Both of those cows shifted their weight from one rear leg to the other, lowing softly with the discomfort of their udders and concern for their offspring. I turned back to the calves. I had my work cut out for me.

❖

Maureen had come up to the barn area from the house, a plastic poncho covering her round figure against the misting rain and chill. She offered me a ceramic cup of hot, steaming coffee, which I accepted readily. I was going to be a while in the damp outdoors, administering treatment to these calves. The hot coffee would help make the experience more bearable.

From the description of the calves Archie had given me over the phone, I figured dehydration would undoubtedly be part of the calves' problems, and I had loaded a case of liter bags of intravenous fluids into my truck. I went to the pickup to set up an IV set for each calf. I rigged three bags with tubing, selected a catheter for each calf, and got my battery-powered hair clippers out. I returned to the tarp-draped calves and shaved a patch of hair from the neck of each calf, just over the jugular vein. After a quick scrub to the shaved area, it was time to set the catheters. The weakest calf was most in need of the life-saving fluids, but her condition was so poor, any attempt to try to save her life was probably futile. I looked up at Archie. He was kneeling down next to the calf with me, waiting to help in any way I asked.

"She's pretty bad, Archie," I began. "It may be just a waste of my time and your money to try to save her."

Bad as I knew that sounded, I considered it wrong not warn an owner of the costs about to be incurred and the likelihood of success. As a veterinarian and also as a compassionate human being, I hated to see an animal suffer and die needlessly, but I also understood the economics of cattle raising.

Archie pressed his lips tightly in thought. His eyes scanned the ailing calf, taking in her labored breathing and sad condition. He placed a hand on her cold shoulder.

"Well," he said carefully, "with treatment she might die anyway. But without treatment, she'll die for sure. If she lives, I might be able to make up the cost later. If she dies, it's just a lesson learned."

He sat back on his heels. "Go ahead and treat her," he said firmly. "We gotta give her the chance."

I nodded and carefully set the IV catheter into the jugular vein. Within minutes, the fluids were rushing down the plastic tubing from the bag into the calf's system. I handed the bag to Maureen to hold while I set the catheters in the neck veins of the other two calves, with Archie's help.

In short order, we had fluids running to the three calves. Maureen held up the two bags with lines leading to the sicker calves, while Archie held the third bag aloft with one hand, the other holding the rowdy bull calf to prevent it from struggling to leave. I prepared antibiotics for injection into the bags of fluids. It wasn't long before the first calf's bag was almost empty.

"We'll probably end up giving her three liters," I told the Drummonds, indicating the first calf. I pushed the liquid antibiotic into each of the bags of IV fluids. "I think two liters will be good for this calf, and one will be sufficient for Bronco Billy there."

As I stepped back from that procedure, I noticed Maureen grimace in discomfort from holding the two bags of fluids aloft. I took one from her, and she smiled gratefully.

"Sure would be good to have an IV stand," I jokingly said, looking around at the treeless terrain.

A light sparkled in Maureen's eyes.

"We could use the tractor," she said, pointing toward a large, green machine parked across the field. It had a front-end loader, plus a hay spear on the back. "We can hang the bags on the loader."

"That's a great idea," Archie said, bouncing to his feet and handing his wife the bag he'd been holding high over his calf. "I'll go get it."

He trotted across the field toward the tractor and climbed into the cab. In a minute, the tractor roared to life, farting a plume of exhaust into the chilly air. It bucked in place as Archie popped it into gear. He angled the machine toward us, raising the front bucket high as he approached.

The two sicker calves paid no heed to the approaching mechanical monster. The third, livelier calf made a half-hearted attempt to rise up under my steadying hand on his withers, before settling down into the hay again. The great diesel tractor blatted its way over to us, looming huge and smelling of fuel and oil. The bucket dropped slowly until the lip hovered at about shoulder height.

Cutting the tractor engine, Archie climbed down out of the cab and came around to scrutinize the placement of the machine. Satisfied, he took one of the bags of IV fluids and carefully hooked the handle of it on one of the prongs that protruded from the bucket. As it swayed gently, he took another bag and did the same thing, while I hung up the third bag.

Now we had three calves lying side-by-side, plastic tubing stretching from their necks to the IV bags that swung from the lip of a huge machine as it stood with authority over us. Freed from holding the bags, Maureen rubbed her arms gently to ease their fatigue and then gathered up our coffee mugs. Archie settled down next to the strongest calf, and I went to prepare some medication to leave for treatment of the calves over the next few days.

Maureen said she would be back in a minute with fresh coffee. She took off in a hurried walk for the house. Archie assessed the arrangement of tarps and then began to rearrange the top tarp, so that in a few minutes he had suspended the tarp from the raised arms of the front-end loader. Now we could sit under the cover, out of the misting rain, while tending the calves.

I had just slowed the administration rates of the fluids, after replacing the empty bags with new ones, when the weakest calf showed her first response to the treatment. As the fluids had coursed into her, rehydrating her body cells, she had taken on a "fuller" look; the desiccated appearance of her body fading. As we watched, her neck relaxed and her eyes, which had been rolled up under the lids, descended to allow the irises to show. Her gasping breath became less labored. She blinked.

"Doc?" Archie asked. "Does that calf look a little better?"

"She does," I confirmed. "We might have something to work with yet." With care, I repositioned the calf's legs, so that they folded under her, and set her up on her chest. Her head, now loosely hung on her neck, swiveled to her flank and nestled there. Her breathing eased, and she appeared to sleep.

The second calf had responded well to the fluid therapy and sat up strongly, eyes bright and alert. When the mother cow, seeing her calf move, lowed gently, the calf bleated in return. This began an anxious barrage of lows and moos from the cows, answered with surprisingly loud bellows from the two stronger calves. Neither calf attempted to stand, however, and after a minute or so, the cows quieted, continuing their worried vigil in silence.

Archie excused himself for a moment and trotted down the slope toward the house. He passed his wife as she made her return trip with a thermos of hot coffee. They exchanged quiet words before continuing on their paths. Maureen handed me a clean cup, uncapped the thermos, and filled the cup with black, aromatic brew. We silently studied the three patients.

"Those two look good," Maureen observed, nodding at the stronger calves, "and I never would have thought that little one would make it."

We watched as the small heifer began to shiver, her body responding to the fluids beginning to warm up her system. I knelt down and checked her rectal temperature. At 97 degrees, it was still well below the normal calf temperature of 102, but definitely on the rise. I smiled up at Maureen.

"She's coming around," I said.

Archie returned from the house shortly, toting three folding camp chairs. We each took one and settled under the tarp to keep an eye on the patients, sipping our coffee and making small talk about weather, the price of cattle, pasture maintenance, and other ranch topics.

The big gray bull calf's IV had run dry. He was attempting to stand up, having thrust his butt into the air, one front leg thrown forward. In another second, he had gained all four feet. He bellowed strongly at his mother, who answered loudly in return. The other two cows began to bawl at their calves, hoping for an answer. The bigger heifer bleated alertly and also attempted to rise. I hurried to remove the IV catheter from the bull calf. No sooner did I have it free of his vein than he bucked strongly under our hands and surged toward his mother. We let him go. He trotted to her and began nursing enthusiastically. The cow ran her long, raspy tongue over his back. He suckled noisily, his tail flapping back and forth with vigor. We grinned.

I removed the IV from the bigger heifer, and Archie and I encouraged her to stand. With a heave, she rose to all four feet. She stood shaking a few minutes before calling to her mother. The cow, anxious to be nursed and relieved of the milk engorging her udder, bellowed happily. The calf staggered out from under the tarp toward her. Like a newborn, she prodded along her mother's side and flank, seeking the udder, which the cow presented impatiently. The cow gasped in alarm when the calf found the udder and butted it, but she didn't kick at the calf. She allowed the calf to fumble and find the teat. So eager to be nursed was she that great streams of milk began to run from her udder. What a look of relief she assumed as the calf found the teat and began to nurse, first hesitantly, then deeply and eagerly.

We turned our attention to the last calf, still lying in the hay, an IV dripping clear, antibiotic-laden fluid into her veins. The mother cow, hearing the wet suckling of the other two calves, again lowed at her calf, encouraging it to live. I evaluated the cow's condition from my position under the tarp.

"We need to get some of that milk off that cow's udder," I told Archie. "You think we can get her in the pen?"

"We can try," he answered, heaving to his feet and heading for the barn. "She'll usually follow a feed bucket."

He returned in a couple of minutes carrying a galvanized bucket half filled with range cubes. When the cow heard the cubes rattle in the bucket, she immediately turned her attention from her calf to the bucket. All her attention focused on the metal container. She glanced back at her calf, seemed to note that it did not move or appear in any danger, and stretched her head out to the bucket. Archie fed her a single cube from his hand. The cow wrapped her tongue around it, took it from him, and chewed it thoughtfully. With a quick flick of her ear toward her calf, she began to walk to Archie. He carefully walked backward, luring the cow into the pen next to the barn. As they passed through the gate, I slipped up and closed it behind the cow. She turned and looked back toward her calf and lowed, long and low. When the calf did not answer, she seemed to shrug and then once again sought out the food-giving bucket.

Archie gave her another cube out of his hand, then turned and walked to the end of the pen, the cow following calmly behind him. He started down the long alleyway of the gathering chute. With just a moment's hesitation, the cow went down the chute behind him. This easy penning was certainly an advantage of working with gentle cattle that had no fear of their human handlers. I placed a bar behind her, to keep her from backing out of the chute. In no time, Archie had lured her into the squeeze chute. Since the cow was cooperative and not struggling, we elected to forgo catching her head in the head gate. We would milk her as she stood in the chute.

Her bag was tight and sore, but except for a half-hearted kick, the cow did not object to me cleaning her teats, applying a little skin-softening udder balm, and milking about a gallon of milk from her. As I finished up, the cow stood quietly, eyes half closed in a daze of relief from the painful pressure. Archie opened the chute to release her from its confines. He poured the rest of the cubes out on the ground for her to eat. I went back to see how the calf was faring.

I was amazed to see the heifer sitting up on her own, her eyes open and liquid again from the fluid therapy, her ears pitched forward in alertness. She looked like she had gained thirty pounds, all of it plumping her skin and giving her hair a shine. Maureen sat in her chair, coffee cup in one hand, the other resting on the calf's withers.

"She tried to get up," she reported happily, "only she was too weak, and I made her stay still. I think she'll make it, don't you?"

I had to agree. What a couple of hours ago had been a dried-up shell of a creature was now vibrating with life. I carefully removed the IV catheter, the fluid bag having emptied out. As I stepped out from under the tarp, a dazzling ray of sunshine split the cloudy sky and sent bright light spilling across the ground. Everything that a moment before had been cloaked in mist and grayness sparkled in the brightness with watery jewels and color. A large patch of blue sky blossomed; clouds changed from monochrome gray to brilliant white. Blades of green grass seemed to spring suddenly from the mud, giving a fresh, vibrant color to the ground. Flashes of blue and rusty red appeared along the fencerow, as eastern bluebirds, cheered by the appearance of the sun, made their presence known with gleeful chirping. A flock of crows, cawing raucously, rose from the field beyond, their wings flashing purple-black in the new sun. A gentle breeze brushed over the emerging grass, bringing the smell of the coming spring. I breathed deeply. I felt completely satisfied with my life at that moment.

Archie returned to the calf, grinning in surprised joy at her obvious return to the living. With a flourish he threw the tarp up and back, so that the warming sunshine could fall on the heifer. Her coat, not so long ago dry and lifeless, now glowed, the red of it gleaming in the light. She suddenly bleated, long and loud. The mother cow, still scooping up the range cubes, jerked her head up in surprise at the sound of her calf, cubes raining from her gaping mouth. She bellowed excitedly and trotted toward us. With great snuffling breaths, she checked her offspring over stem to stern.

The heifer, invigorated, struggled to gain her feet. Archie and I sprang to her aid, helping her remain upright as she tottered toward the anxious cow. Trembling from the effort, the calf, weakened by her ordeal, nuzzled her mother's flank for the udder. The cow stood rock-still, waiting for the calf's tongue to wrap around one of the teats. It was wonderful to hear the wet sound of suckling, at first slow and weak, then stronger and faster. After just a short time, we were able to remove our steadying hands from the heifer. She continued to suckle vigorously for several minutes before becoming exhausted from the effort. She panted, her belly full. After appearing to think about the situation, she slowly turned and staggered back to the tarp, folded her legs up, and collapsed into the hay. This time when she folded her head around to her flank, it was in deep sleep, not the stupor of oncoming death.

The Drummonds and I grinned at each other in pleasure at the sight. What started out as a cold, misty day with death in the forecast ended in a sun-filled afternoon with three calves bounding in life, each with a great chance of survival. Even the smell of sickness had dissipated on the slight breeze that fluttered the edge of the tarp and ruffled the shiny red hairs of the calf. I began to pick up the used fluid bags and other equipment. It was time to head back to town.

I dropped the trash into the truck's disposal can and looked back at the calf. Bright, long, low beams of late-afternoon sunlight made the drops of rain and little puddles of water on the ground glitter. The cow stood contently over her calf, chewing the range cubes being fed to her by Maureen, who had fetched the feed off the ground. Archie worked to remove the protecting tarp, no longer needed, from the front of his tractor. It was a very good picture.

❖

As I stood by my truck in the warming sunshine, watching the revived calf, hearing the twitter of birds out seeking seeds for dinner, listening to the grinding of the cow's teeth on her feed, I knew why I did what I did for a living. It was for moments like this. This peaceful, bucolic scene of contented cows and satisfied owners. This picture of life after such a close brush with death. This result of my education and dedication to life.

I breathed in deeply of the crisp, cool winter air and sighed with contentment. I was profoundly grateful to the people like the Drummonds, who called upon me and trusted me to help them with their animals. The will to live and remarkable ability to rebound in creatures such as these calves was simply amazing. I was delighted to be a party to it all. I was happy. At that moment, I couldn't think of any better way to earn a living.

Dr. Russell and the
State Trooper

Why should man expect his prayer for mercy to be heard by what
is above him when he shows no mercy to what is under him?
— Pierre Troubetzkoy

Quite a bit of my experience with cattle was gained while working as an assistant and technician for other veterinarians in the
years before I went to veterinary college myself. Some of those
times I remember fondly. Others occasionally spring unbidden
from my memory storage boxes, and I relive the event in all its
color and sound and odor and texture. Sometimes that's good.
Sometimes, it's not so good.

❖

Dr. Frank A. Russell was a tall, lean young veterinarian who came
to work at the Twin City Animal Hospital in 1974. He had been
hired as an associate to the owner-partners, Dr. Francis N.
McClellen and Dr. Greg L. Roberts, my bosses. I had been hired
there only a few months earlier as a veterinary assistant/techni-
cian. My duties included helping with cases, cleaning, inventory,
and often working the front desk. Most Sundays found me in the
kennels, cleaning cages and feeding the animals that were board-

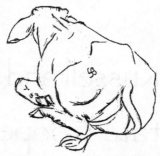

ing there or caring for any patients held over the weekend. I loved my job. Veterinary college was still far into my future.

When Dr. Russell came on board, it took me awhile to adjust to having three people to answer to, to assist, and to clean up after. I did all right. I lived for the days when I was called upon by one of them to jump into a pickup and accompany him on a ranch call. I loved being out in the country, working with the horses and cattle on the ranches that used the Twin City veterinarians. I know I learned volumes watching these men work, and I couldn't wait to get to work every morning, to see what else might be happening in the intriguing world of veterinary medicine.

Dr. Russell came in one freezing Sunday morning while I was at the hospital cleaning up after the boarding dogs and cats. He'd come to stock his truck with supplies before heading out on a calf delivery call. He asked me if I wanted to go along. I had not assisted Dr. Russell on a cattle job at that point, and I jumped at the chance.

We loaded into his little Chevy S10 and off we went to Thompson, a small community about fifteen miles from the hospital. Our patient turned out to be an undersized heifer trying to deliver an oversized calf. As Dr. McClellen would have said, "A calf trying to have a cow."

Mr. Haverty had the cow in a pen that was fortunately under a roof, considering the stiff, cold wind blowing from the north. Nonetheless, due to recent rains, puddles of iced-over water dotted the soggy ground. The cow had lain down before we got there and was straining half-heartedly, a steaming puddle of amniotic fluid on the ground beneath her tail. Two white hooves peeked from her vagina as she strained and disappeared again when she relaxed. Mr. Haverty had thoughtfully stockpiled a stack of empty paper feed sacks to place on the ground behind the downed heifer to give Dr. Russell a somewhat dry area on which to kneel while he worked.

Dr. Russell reluctantly removed his coat while I fetched warm water in the gallon jugs we'd brought with us, as well as the OB sleeves and soap. He was already shivering in the cold air as he slid the crackling plastic gloves on one at a time. He soaped up and then rubbed his hands and arms vigorously, working to raise a lather in the cold air.

"I almost can't wait to get to work," he said jokingly. "At least it'll be warm inside the cow."

That was one of the good things I was to learn about calf deliveries on cold days. Once you went to work inside the huge, warm body of the cow, you didn't even notice how cold it was outside. As you strained and sweated from the exertion of working whilst armpit-deep in a cow, observers could be freezing as they waited to help.

Dr. Russell knelt on a clean paper feed sack behind the little heifer. His initial exam was done quickly. He sat back on his heels and looked up at Mr. Haverty, who stood near the fence with his coat collar turned up against the wind, his hat pulled down firmly on his head.

"The calf is dead," Dr. Russell informed him. "The head's turned back. We're going to have to cut the calf up to get it out."

"What's that going to cost me?" asked Mr. Haverty.

It wasn't an uncommon question. The commercial raising of calves for the beef market was not a high-paying career. The decision to keep or sell a breeding cow was based on economics. If her value as a brood animal that would produce calves for sale was greater than the expense of fixing a problem, then a rancher would gamble on a veterinarian's skill to correct the problem. If the expense outweighed the cow's value, in many instances the cow's life was terminated or she was sold at a sale barn as quickly as possible.

The profit in cattle production can be so marginal that many ranchers will sell a problem cow rather than risk her costing him more later on. The sale barns see many cows brought to market with histories of problems such as vaginal or uterine prolapse, a bad udder, dystocia—anything that might compromise her ability to reproduce and/or raise a calf. Even a non-reproductive problem, such as lameness, can seriously affect a cow's ability to get around and graze, carry a calf to term, or keep up with the herd. A sick or lame cow is a liability and will be sold quickly to lessen her drag on the finances of the ranch.

I've heard many a rancher say it costs as much to feed a bad cow as it does to feed a good cow, so might as well only feed the good ones. In actuality, a bad cow costs more.

So, when Mr. Haverty asked the cost of removing the dead calf from the cow, he had already calculated the cow's worth as she lay on the ground before him, which was nothing, against her potential if the vet was able to save her. He needed to know if any further expenditure would recoup his losses. If the cow could be saved, he could sell her after a couple months to make up the cost of the procedure. If she could not only be saved but also salvaged as a breeding animal, the veterinary costs would be an investment for future profits.

Dr. Russell closed his eyes and mentally added up the cost of the work to be done. He opened them and faced Mr. Haverty.

"I can get the calf out in one of two ways," he said. "We could do a C-section. It would be fast and the cow would probably recover fine from the surgery, but you'd have to sell her. Her chances of having a calf without a problem later might not be good. If I cut the calf up, what's called a fetotomy, the cow would have a better chance of having calves again."

He stopped, waiting for Mr. Haverty to think over what he'd just told him. Then he added, "The C-Section would cost you about $100. The fetotomy won't be as much, and the risk is less to the cow."

Mr. Haverty rubbed his chin, staring down at his little cow, which grunted as she strained against the twisted calf inside her. When he said nothing, Dr. Russell spoke again.

"This is her first calf," he said. "She's in good shape now, and she's a nice-looking cow. I'd bet she'd go on to make you a good cow. But if you want to sell her anyway, if we did a C-section and she went to sale, you'd just get slaughter prices when they saw her incision. If we do the fetotomy, she'd probably bring a better price at the barn."

Mr. Haverty nodded in understanding.

"If we don't do anything, she dies," he mused. He made up his mind then. "Do it," he said. "If you can get it out without doing a C-section, do it."

Boy, was I excited. Though a bit disappointed that I wouldn't get to see a C-section on a cow, something I'd never witnessed, I'd never seen a fetotomy done, either. I loped alongside Dr. Russell back to the truck, to help get the equipment he would need to do the job. Armed with the instruments, we hurried back to help the cow.

The job turned out to be messier than anything I had anticipated. Dr. Russell stopped early on to remove his sweatshirt. Not only was he warmed from the exertion of the job, but he also didn't want to get his clothes any nastier than necessary. He resumed work with just a T-shirt to cover his torso. Mr. Haverty kept busy, replacing the wet and dirty feed sacks on the ground behind the cow with clean ones, as needed.

Though the calf was dead before the procedure began, it was still fresh and the blood had not clotted in its veins. Bright red blood washed over the doctor's arms as he worked. He had to remove the calf's head and neck, severing it from the body with a long, serrated wire run through the fetotome, the metal tube that prevented injury to the cow.

Once the head and neck were separated from the calf's body and removed, Dr. Russell was able to deliver the rest of the calf with only moderate effort. Chains were applied to the front limbs. I worked the lever of the calf puller, following Dr. Russell's instructions, to slowly draw the fetus out of the cow.

With the remains of the calf delivered, Dr. Russell removed the already loosened afterbirth from the cow. He placed two antiseptic boluses in her uterus to ward off infection. A penicillin injection followed. While we carried our equipment back to the truck, the cow, as if suddenly aware she was no longer burdened with the dead calf, stood up. Mr. Haverty was very pleased with the results of Dr. Russell's efforts, and he quickly wrote a check.

When Dr. Russell turned back to the pickup, shivering in the cold, I held up his coat to him. He started to take it, but then looked down at his T-shirt and arms, now soaked with blood and birth fluids.

"That's a new coat," he said. "I don't want to get this stuff all over it. I won't put it on. I'll just turn up the heater in the truck and drive back fast."

I held onto the outerwear. He folded his long legs up as he got into the driver's seat. I ran around and jumped into the passenger seat. We waved to Mr. Haverty as he held the gate for our departure. Dr. Russell cranked the heater knob of the truck over to full power, shivering violently as the moisture on his body and clothes cooled in the frigid winter air. He threw the truck into gear, and we bumped down the ranch lane to the highway. Traffic was minimal on this early Sunday morning, and Dr. Russell jammed the accelerator to the floorboard. The little pickup jumped, screaming, and took off at high speed.

I just held on to my seat, clutching the doctor's coat in my lap. The heater was noisily cranking out warm air, and Dr. Russell was leaning over the steering wheel, still shivering. Suddenly, he sat up, staring into the rearview mirror.

"Uh-oh," he said, taking his foot from the accelerator.

I twisted around and looked out the back window. Roaring up behind our pickup was a state trooper's black-and-white car, the red and blue lights on the top flashing. The siren was just audible over the noise of the truck's raging engine and heater fan. As the engine slowed, we could clearly hear the shrill whining of the sirens. Dr. Russell let the truck slow and drifted it to the road's shoulder.

"How fast were you going?" I asked, as the truck bumped over the rough gravel surface of the shoulder.

"I don't know. About eighty, I guess," he said, watching the rearview mirror as the trooper stopped behind us. The siren's wail wound down, but the red and blue lights continued to flicker, rotating their colors through the rear window of the truck. The speed limit on that stretch of highway was 65 mph. If Dr. Russell had been doing 80 mph, then we'd been speeding, and properly caught at it, too.

"Maybe I can explain it to him," Dr. Russell said. He was agitated, nervous. "Maybe if I explain we just finished a calf delivery, and I wanted to get back fast because I was cold." Without giving me a chance to give my opinion, he wrenched the door handle and pushed the door open.

I glanced back at the officer, who was not looking toward our vehicle. He'd gotten out of his car and was bending back in, apparently to get his ticket book. Dr. Russell had leaped out of the truck and was taking long strides toward him.

The officer was just straightening up and placing his Smokey hat on his head when he looked up and saw the rapidly approaching man. He started, his face collapsing with shock and fear. He dropped his ticket book onto the pavement. He stumbled backwards, clawing at his holster with both hands but unable to unbuckle the flap.

I stared, gape-mouthed. I could see what he could see—a tall, T-shirted man covered with blood almost running toward him. Combined with the intense look in his eyes and the determined set of his chin, Dr. Russell must have looked like a mass murderer just off a slaughter binge and now bent on annihilating the officer too.

My immediate thought was, *Oh, my Lord, I'm going to see a man get shot.* I was sure that any second the officer would get his gun free of the holster. I would see him crouch slightly, both hands gripping the gun. I would hear him yell "Halt!" Only Dr. Russell wouldn't understand and wouldn't halt. After all, he was just a cold, dirty veterinarian trying to get home fast to clean up and get warm. He just wanted to hurry over and explain the situation to the trooper and go home. The officer wouldn't know that.

Dr. Russell would keep up his rapid advance toward the officer, unaware of the mortal danger he was in. The officer would yell "Halt!" one more time. He would squeeze his eyes shut, his mouth closed so tight his lips would be thin, tense lines. Then he would fire his weapon. It would be horrible. Dr. Russell would be thrown backwards, arms up, his blood bright and wet as it gushed and covered the stains of the calf's blood already drying on his T-shirt. I would be screaming by that time, unable to move. Or maybe I would be screaming while tearing off the truck's door to get out and help my fallen boss. Either way, I would be screaming. I was going to have to start screaming for real any second. Oh, my Lord, I was going to see a man get *shot*!

Thank God, the scenario in my head did not play out there on the highway on that cold Sunday morning.

As the obviously frightened officer backpedaled, fumbling for his weapon, Dr. Russell threw up his hands and started talking. I could barely hear his voice over the rumble of the truck's engine and the loud hum of the heater fan. I could see the officer, his face blanched white, nodding vigorously, fingers clenching and unclenching over his holster. I could see that he had unsnapped the flap on the holster. I could see the gun was half out of the holster, too. Dr. Russell was talking loudly, flapping his hands as he explained why he was speeding. The officer kept nodding his head rapidly and waved Dr. Russell away.

As Dr. Russell gave the officer a thumbs-up and turned back to the pickup, I watched as the trooper slumped, knees buckled, against the side of his car. As Dr. Russell hustled back to the pickup, grinning, I saw the officer, color creeping back into his cheeks, blow out a long breath, white in the cold air, and stagger upright. He pulled his open car door back a little more, looked down briefly, and got into the car. I wondered if he was checking his pants for wetness. I wondered if he would report the incident back at the station.

Dr. Russell flung his long body into the driver's seat, slammed his door, and threw the shifter into first gear. He popped the clutch, sending the little Chevy hopping down the highway.

"He let me go with just a warning," he said, totally unaware of the dramatic scene I had witnessed, partly real, partly imagined.

"He almost shot you," I gravely informed him. The truck swerved sharply. I looked quickly back toward the trooper. His car had not moved. The lights were still flashing round and round, red-blue-red-blue.

"What?" Dr. Russell squeaked, jerking his head around to stare at me.

"He almost shot you," I repeated. "Lucky for you, he couldn't get his gun out of his holster."

"Why was he going to shoot me?" Dr. Russell's voice had gone an octave higher than normal, with a little tremor making it almost musical in quality.

"Look at yourself," I told him. "He probably thought you had just murdered a bunch of people and he was next."

Puzzled, he glanced down at his shirt front. His eyes widened and his mouth fell open in an O. The truck swerved a little again. He plucked at his messy shirt with the fingers of his right hand, his left hand on the steering wheel, trying to hold the truck in the correct highway lane. I could see the blood draining from his face as he realized what I said was true, leaving it even whiter in contrast to the bloody T-shirt.

❖

Neither one of us said another word on the way to the hospital. I don't know if Dr. Russell ever told the other two veterinarians what happened on that drive back from a bloody calf delivery. I never mentioned it. I do know that Dr. Russell never left on a call after that without a clean shirt to change into. And I don't believe he ever, ever got a ticket for speeding.

Mr. Bryan's Ragged Little Heifer

*Because the heart beats under a covering of hair, of fur,
feathers, or wings, it is, for that reason, to be of no account?*
—Jean Paul Richter

Cattle ranching is an economic venture, for the most part. While
some folks get a few cows to putter around with and use on their
tax forms, raising cattle for a living is time-consuming hard work,
and ranchers often barely break even at the end of the year.
Calves are generally weaned and sold as soon as possible. Good
heifers might be kept back to replace cows that have been
removed from the herd. Aged or otherwise poor-producing cows
are usually culled from the herd and sold before they become too
much of a liability.

❖

Ronald Bryan kept a large herd of Black Angus cows with a Hereford bull. The cross between the two breeds resulted in a com-
mercially popular calf known as a black baldy, an animal with a
black body and a white face. The baldy steers and heifers were
usually the best sellers to feedlot buyers, and they paid good
money to load their trucks with the white-faced calves. Mr. Bryan.

144

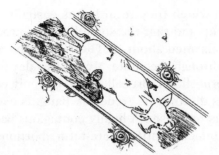

generally sold all the calves produced in his commercial herd, including all the heifers.

Mr. Bryan also kept another herd comprised of registered Black Angus cows and a good Angus bull. This herd, smaller than his commercial one, produced the replacement heifers he put into his commercial herd as the cows aged, lost production, or were otherwise culled.

I received a call one day from Mr. Bryan to come to his ranch to vaccinate the purebred Angus heifers he'd decided to keep as replacements. He had about thirty head, just five months old, and we set a date for the vaccinations.

The day dawned a beautiful fall morning. Leaves had turned to golds and reds, yellows and browns. The air was crisp and clean, the sky a uniform, brilliant blue. It was a fine day to work cattle.

Mr. Bryan was a calm, easy-going man around his cows, and the peace he radiated as he went about his work was reflected in the cattle's demeanor. Usually when I went to work cows for him, he was the only one there to do the sorting and moving of the cattle. He was so relaxed in his job that the cattle rarely gave him any trouble.

When I arrived at the ranch, the heifers were standing quietly in the holding pen. I climbed out of my pickup. Mr. Bryan strode over, and we shook hands solemnly. I turned to survey the heifers in the pen.

They were a beautifully uniform group, each calf the same size and shape as the next. They were fat and slick, obviously well fed and tended. They all had glossy black coats and shiny black eyes with which they regarded us casually. They knew something was up and that the something involved them, but they were not alarmed about it. They would be a nice, easy group to guide through the chute. My job this day was to vaccinate them for brucellosis. Brucellosis, commonly called Bang's Disease after its discoverer, Frederick Bang, is caused by the *Brucella abortus* organism. A highly contagious bacterium, its worst effect on infected cattle is late-term abortions in susceptible cows.

Prevention of the disease involves vaccinating heifer calves when they are between the ages of four and twelve months. Brucella organisms can infect humans, causing symptoms known as "undulant fever" in the United States and by different names in other countries. Because humans can contract it, it is a reportable disease, meaning cases of it, human or animal, must be reported to the proper government officials.

At the time I was practicing cattle medicine, brucellosis management and control was a federally and state-regulated operation in Texas. Only a licensed veterinarian could handle the vaccine and vaccinate heifers against the disease. To show they had been officially vaccinated against the disease, a tattoo was applied to the inside of the right ear of each calf. The tattoo indicated the year and the quarter of the year the vaccine was given, as well as having a V-shield emblem in its center. The V-shield meant a licensed veterinarian had administered the vaccine in the proper manner.

Along with the permanent tattoo, an elongated orange metal tag was stapled to the right ear. The orange tag was an individual identification tag for the heifer. The tags were sequentially numbered, one assigned to each calf vaccinated. The numbers were recorded on an official state form, in quadruplicate. One copy was given to the owner, one was stored in the administering veterinarian's files, and two were sent to the state offices of the Texas Animal Health Commission.

As I mixed the vaccine and set out my syringes, needles, tattoo pliers and ink, and the paperwork on a clipboard with a pen to make the necessary notations, I noticed an odd-man-out in the group of calves. Cavorting with one of the black calves at the back of the group was a white-faced red calf. She was much smaller than the black heifers, with a long, rough haircoat that stuck out in all directions. Her hipbones thrust out from her skinny body, in sharp contrast to the robust builds of the other calves. I might not have noticed her at all, small as she was, except for the fact that she was bouncing around merrily, butting the other heifer with the tiny horn nubs sprouting on her head.

I glanced over to Mr. Bryan, intending to ask him about the heifer, but he was occupied setting up the gates of the chute in preparation for starting the heifers down the alleyway. I figured the red heifer was probably just accidentally mixed in with the black calves. She certainly didn't look like any heifer I'd ever seen produced on the Bryan ranch.

The alleyway to the squeeze chute in this set of pens was just long enough to accommodate five calves at one time. That worked out fine for me, as the vaccine needed to be mixed in lots of five doses. While Mr. Bryan was bringing up each group of calves, I could be mixing the next vial of vaccine. It always proved to be an efficient way for us to work.

In a couple of minutes, five of the little heifers started down the chute, one behind the other in an orderly manner. Vaccinating thirty heifers with such good behavior would be a cinch to get done quickly. Mr. Bryan would send a calf into the squeeze chute where I would catch her neck in the head gate.

I vaccinated the first five with ease, the tattoos and ear tags going in with barely a bawl from any of them. After finishing each calf, I released the hold of the head gate on the calf and let her go while Mr. Bryan pushed the next calf forward into the chute. It was going like clockwork.

When we finished with the first five calves, Mr. Bryan walked back to the sorting pen to get another group of five. As I mixed my next vial of vaccine, I noticed the red heifer charging around the pen, kicking up her heels and harassing the black calves. They appeared undisturbed by her bullying and continued to walk sedately toward the chute and down the alleyway. I figured

Mr. Bryan would sort the little renegade out from the group as we worked.

The second group of five heifers were vaccinated and tattooed as easily as the first. Mr. Bryan went back for the third round of calves while I mixed my vaccine and put a new needle on the syringe. I watched out the corner of my eye as the little red heifer tried her best to disrupt the orderliness of the process, but the black heifers chose to ignore her, instead paying attention to the tall rancher who urged them down the chute.

As the sorting pen emptied out with each group of five black heifers moving down the alleyway, the red heifer became a little wilder, a little more frantic in her bucking and carrying on in the pen. She bawled and shook her head menacingly at Mr. Bryan as he moved calmly around the pen. Mr. Bryan continued to ignore her. Each time I looked his way, intending to ask about that heifer, he quickly looked away.

I was beginning to think this little outcast might be an embarrassment to him. Or maybe he was thinking that if he ignored her and just got the black ones to move where he wanted them to, the red one would sort herself out from the herd. Then he could release her to the pasture without worrying about losing the others. Or maybe he intended to keep her in the pen so he could turn her over to the rightful owner whenever he found out who that might be. I sure didn't know, and Mr. Bryan wasn't giving me an opportunity to ask.

We were down to the last group of heifers, four black ones and the feisty little red one. As Mr. Bryan directed the little group into the alleyway, the red calf crowded into the space with the black ones. She was third in line, locked between two black heifers in front and two behind. She was pitching a fit over the confinement, bawling and wiggling fiercely, alternating between trying to barge ahead of the calves in front of her and pushing backwards between the two behind her. The black heifers all ignored her, enduring with grace her wild attempts to escape. Mr. Bryan ignored her. I couldn't ignore her. This bony, shaggy little heifer was showing the world her spirit. She was something.

I vaccinated the first two heifers without a problem. I waited to see if Mr. Bryan would tell me to leave the head gate open, to allow the red heifer to go out.

"Catch her," was all he said when he noticed my questioning look.

As she surged forward into the squeeze chute, I deftly caught her neck in the head gate. She was so much smaller than the other calves she was able to wiggle quite freely in the chute. She bawled and fought the restraint.

Once again I looked for direction from Mr. Bryan. What did he want me to do with this calf?

In answer he diverted his eyes toward the last two calves in the alleyway and said quietly, "Vaccinate her."

I looked down at the angry little cow-to-be. She grew still for a moment, reaching out to snuffle my clothing. I leaned over her and gave her the injection in her neck. She sure didn't like that, emitting a squealing bawl in protest. She resented the tattoo application even more, bawling in indignation as I swiped the ink over the deep imprint left in her ear by the instrument. After applying the orange ear tag, I glanced up to Mr. Bryan again, to see him wave his hand to indicate I should release the calf. I opened the head gate, and she bounded out, kicking once in my direction as she bucked her way over to the other heifers milling around the pen.

Without looking up toward me, Mr. Bryan urged the next heifer into the squeeze chute. We finished up the job in another few minutes. I was curious about the red heifer, but it was apparent that Mr. Bryan didn't want to discuss it. Since it was his business, I let it go.

As I loaded my supplies into the truck and got out the bill box to make out the ticket, Mr. Bryan tidied up the area around his pens. He opened a gate at the far end of the pen the heifers occupied, so that they could return to the pasture beyond. The out-of-place red heifer bounced along with the sedate group of black heifers, a flitting, ragged red contrast to the quietly strolling Angus.

I stood watching the calves leave, still wondering about that little red heifer, when Mr. Bryan spoke.

"I suppose you're wondering about that red nothin' calf," he said. I turned toward him. He was standing easily, his hands thrust into his hip pockets as he watched the calves spread out into the pasture.

"Actually, I am curious," I admitted. "She sure doesn't fit into that group."

"That heifer," he began, shaking his head as if in wonder, while keeping an eye on her retreating tail. "She was born to one of the old commercial cows I keep in the other herd. I don't recall ever getting a red calf out of one of my good black cows before, but here this little scallywag shows up. The cow didn't want it and wouldn't feed it. I couldn't catch a hold of her, and I figured she'd just die in the pasture, give the coyotes a free meal." He shook his head again, as if in amazement. "That little rascal survived by going cow to cow and stealing milk."

Mr. Bryan stopped talking for a moment, placing the fingertips of his right hand on his chin, his eyes going soft as he kept them on his little herd. He turned and looked me in the eye, perhaps for the first time that day.

"Anything that wants to live that much," he stated emphatically, "I'm going to let it. She's always going to have a place in my herd. And if you think I'm a little crazy because I keep her, well then, that's just your problem, not mine."

I smiled broadly.

"No, Mr. Bryan, I don't think you're crazy at all," I told him. "And that's one lucky little heifer out there."

We stood a moment longer, gazing out over the pasture after the calves. Finally, I turned back toward my truck to leave the ranch. Mr. Bryan solemnly saluted in my direction as I pulled out of his gate. I tipped my imaginary hat in his direction in return and continued on my way.

❖

I've thought about Mr. Bryan and his little red calf often over the years. I loved the case, loved that the heifer grew up and eventually calmed down, joining his commercial herd and raising her own little feisty red calves in the years that followed. I loved the proof that there are good people out there who don't look at their cattle merely as a means to make a living, but who regard their charges as sentient creatures with their own minds and hearts, people like Mr. Bryan who are not afraid to honor the animal for what she is—an individual with a will to keep on going in spite of everything against her.

This little heifer survived because of her spirit and determination. In her favor, definitely, was her owner, a man who gave her the chance to live and didn't hold her rowdiness against her, but rather saw it as an asset. In return, the heifer matured, gentled down, and became a contributing member of the herd. I couldn't come up with a better ending to a story if I tried.

Part 5

People and Cows

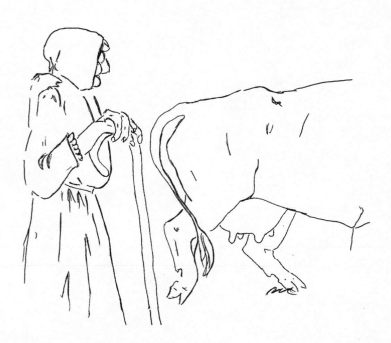

Little Henry's Bloated Cow

Until he extends the circle of compassion to all living things,
man will not himself find peace.
—Albert Schweitzer

Convincing some of the older ranchers that I was capable of doing what was traditionally considered a "man's job" wasn't always easy. Many times I ended up as the veterinarian doing cow work out on a ranch simply because the cowman was desperate for help and I represented the last-ditch effort to save a dying animal. It certainly wasn't a very satisfying reason to be chosen to administer medical aid to a cow. However, after a successful calf delivery or miraculous "cure" of a downer cow, I would often become the veterinarian of choice the next time the rancher needed qualified medical help.

It was humorous, though somewhat irritating, to have some old rancher assume I couldn't do a job because he thought I was too weak. This notion often came from a man whose body was so bent and broken with age that he could barely shuffle over to the pen to watch the work being done.

The work was hard, no doubt about it, but when you come right to the gist of the matter, if a cow doesn't want a person to handle her, regardless of that person's size or strength, it isn't going to happen without a fight. One-hundred-and-fifty pounds of

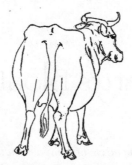

human against a thousand pounds of upset bovine is no contest. That's why cattle chutes and head gates, stout ropes and horses have a place in cattle ranching, and always will.

These things are used to keep cattlemen safe and to give them the leverage they need to handle the cattle. They work just as well for a woman as for a man. Knowing when and how to apply leverage came in handy in a situation I faced early one morning when I got a call-out to look at a downer cow.

❖

The rancher, Little Henry Knight, had gone to his pasture to feed his cattle and had found a cow lying on its side, bloated and unable to rise. He and his two brothers had not even been able to get the cow into the normal resting position of sitting on her chest.

Any cow can bloat, but a cow lying flat on her side is always in grave danger of bloating. In that position, the ingesta in her rumen—the second of a cow's four "stomachs" but more like a huge fermentation vat—moves and covers the esophagus opening. The gases produced by the fermentation cannot escape out the cow's mouth as a belch.

Belching is a highly desirable and necessary result of a cow's somewhat complex digestive process. If a cow doesn't belch the gases produced in her rumen, they accumulate and cause it to balloon to enormous proportions. The bloated rumen then puts pressure on other internal organs, including the heart, lungs, and blood vessels. This pressure will result in the death of the cow if not corrected.

The panic in Little Henry's voice as he reported this emergency indicated he was well aware of the consequences of a cow being down and bloated. He'd had a cow go down once before and die soon thereafter. He wanted me out there as soon as possible.

❖

I hopped in my truck and drove like a fury to the ranch. A young boy was at the gate holding it open for me, so I could drive into the pasture without stopping. He pointed into the distance, and far out in the pasture on a little knoll was a hay ring, a tractor, and three large men. I drove over the bumpy ground to the group.

As I approached, I could see a hugely bloated black cow on her left side, head thrown back and tongue out as she gasped for breath. Her eyes bugged from their sockets with the effort of her breathing. Her upper legs were elevated from the ground and slightly spread, due to her distended abdomen. The skin of her belly was stretched taut and hard. The three men stood in a circle around her, regarding her with a mixture of pity and frustration. I turned off the truck's motor and got out.

Little Henry stepped forward. The man had been named after his father, Henry Knight, Sr. Rather than being called Hank or Henry Jr. as a child, he'd been tagged with Little Henry, and the moniker stayed with him into adulthood. His nickname belied his size. He was enormous. He was built like a young bull and was sober in expression. He looked powerful enough to pick the cow up unassisted and set her on her feet. I felt small and puny next to his bulk. His forearm looked bigger around than my thigh, and at 140 pounds, I wasn't a skinny gal.

We shook hands. My hand completely disappeared inside his clasp, and I felt a momentary spiraling of fear, wondering if he would accidentally crush it. Although he was obviously capable of doing so, his handshake was firm yet gentle.

"I hope you can help us," Little Henry intoned in a soft voice that contradicted the power of his body. "My brothers and I couldn't get the cow up. She's too sick to stand."

I turned my focus on the cow. Her neck was arched back and her breathing was ragged. She appeared to beseech the humans who surrounded her to either help her or finish her off. She knew she was dying.

I surveyed the situation. The cow, while monstrously bloated, was not herself a large cow, but rather a smallish Angus cross. She was lying right up beside the hay ring, a round, metal-pipe contraption about eight feet in diameter, built to surround a half-ton round bale of hay and protect it from being trampled by the cattle it is meant to feed. The cow's feet were slightly uphill, and the two legs on the ground appeared to be wedged under the hay ring. From the signs around her, I knew the cow had struggled for a while before the bloat caused her to concentrate her efforts solely on breathing. Without assistance, this cow was doomed.

I instructed the men to move the hay ring, if they could. Together, Little Henry and his two equally well-built brothers lifted the hay ring off the round bale and set it out of the way. With her feet freed, the cow was still unable to move. She offered no attempt to right herself.

"We need to flip her over," I said. "Her feet are uphill; we need to move her so they're downhill to give her a better chance of getting up."

Little Henry, hands on hips, gave me a slightly condescending look.

"We tried," he said. "Ain't no way we can move her. We were just fixin' to put a chain on her and drag her out with the tractor."

"There's no need for that," I assured him. "We can flip her over without it."

"How?" Little Henry asked, crossing his massive arms over his chest and shaking his head sadly at my ignorance.

"Like this," I said and stepped forward to the cow.

I reached down and grabbed the fetlock of the uppermost front leg. I pulled up, so that the leg was sticking straight up in the air, and continued to bring the leg over. The leverage action gently rotated the cow onto her back, and with a little extra effort on my part, the cow continued to roll until she flopped down on her right side. Her feet were now downhill from her body.

There's a funny thing that often happens with cows when they're turned over. It's like their entire world changes and shifts focus. That's what happened with Little Henry's cow. Suddenly, her outlook on life rearranged itself, and she decided maybe she wasn't dying after all. With her feet pointed downhill, rolling up into a sternal position was easy. She popped up onto her chest, extended her neck and belched mightily, the gas trapped in her rumen having found escape up the now unobstructed esophagus. She took a deep, cleansing breath and belched again.

I glanced up at Little Henry. He and his two brothers were staring, slack-jawed, at the cow. The cow belched again, long, rumbling, and smelling of wet hay. Her rotund belly deflated remarkably as we watched. This was one cow I would not have to deflate with a stomach tube or trocar. She was getting the job done herself.

All three of the men moved their dumbfounded gazes from the deflating cow over to me. As one, and with what appeared to be a great deal of respect, all of them took a giant step backward, away from me.

For a split second I was puzzled by their behavior, and then I realized what I'd just done. Together, these three burly men had been unable to move the cow an inch. Here I come, a thirty-something-year-old woman and not a body builder by any stretch of the imagination. All I did was reach down, grab a foot, and flip the cow like she was made of papier-mâché. Leverage is cool.

I let the feeling hover over us for a minute or two longer. Satisfied that my Wonder Woman image was firmly implanted in these men's minds, I explained to Little Henry that the cow had apparently lain down next to the hay ring and got her feet stuck under it. Combined with the slight incline of the ground, she was unable to right herself again and had bloated. I felt sure the cow would recover now that she was upright.

Sure enough, while we stood there assessing each other, the cow gave a mighty heave and rose shakily to her rear legs. After a moment, she put first one front foot out and then the other. She stood quietly for a minute and then belched again.

I told Little Henry if he found another cow down, he should do whatever was necessary to get her on her feet or in a chest-sitting position. Either position would delay bloating and allow a veterinarian time to arrive and give whatever treatment might be needed.

❖

It was a satisfying trip. I didn't explain to those nice young men how I'd been able to turn the cow over with minimal strength. I wanted that Wonder Woman mystique to linger a little longer. It just goes to show, though, that a person doesn't have to be built like a brick house in order to do a job. But it certainly helps if you know what you're doing.

Country Folks

If a man aspires towards a righteous life,
his first act of abstinence is from injury to animals.
—Albert Einstein

Veterinary medicine is still considered, in some circles, to be a man's profession. My graduating class was one of the first to have more women than men in it, but the ratio of women to men in all the veterinary schools since then has tipped dramatically in favor of women. That doesn't mean, however, that women no longer have to prove themselves when dealing with the real world, especially in large-animal medicine.

After a couple of years in solo practice, I had developed a reputation as a veterinarian who would come out when no one else was available. Or, maybe, it was a reputation for being foolhardy enough to go out in any situation. Sometimes the weather wasn't agreeable. Sometimes the work wasn't. Often, the client was nobody's favorite. And sometimes I was just the only qualified person in town the particular Sunday afternoon when a cow went into labor and couldn't deliver.

That's the way it was one weekend morning when a call came from what sounded like an elderly man. They had a cow down, and he, his son, and a helpful neighbor from down the road had

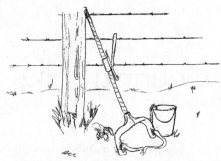

been unable to deliver the calf. Their regular vet was unavailable for the weekend. Could I come out?

Always willing to help an animal in crisis, I agreed to drive out to the ranch. I got the directions and changed into my cow clothes, lightweight coveralls. It was fall, but in our area of the country I didn't need to dress against freezing temperatures. I headed out the door.

It was a long drive out to the ranch, down at least five miles of washed-out sandy road. I crawled along at the maximum speed of a snail. I found the place easily enough and drove up to the house. The cow pens were nearby, and in one pen a cream-colored heifer lay flat on her left side, her belly stretched tight with calf. Surrounding her stood three men, appearing to contemplate the heifer's predicament. One was a wizened little old man with a burning cigarette pinched between two fingers of one hand. Another was a large young man who must have been the son. The third was an older gentleman who radiated the aura of a retired white-collar worker. As I stepped out of the truck, I saw the three men exchange grim looks.

By this time in my career, I'd seen that look a thousand times. It said, "Oh, great, a woman. Just when we need a man for the job." I didn't like it, but I was used to getting the look and chose, as usual, to ignore it. The young man approached me first. After exchanging introductions, he cocked his head toward the down cow.

"She's been in labor a long time," he said. "We think the calf's still alive. We couldn't move it."

"Let me have a look at her," I said. "Then we'll decide what to do."

I got my soap, water, gloves, and OB lube and walked over to the prone cow. She was small, maybe 500 pounds, and worn out from her exertions. She had a rope wrapped around her horns, with the other end tied to a stout fence post, presumably to detain her if she chose to jump up and run away. But the most she did was roll her large brown eyes at me and stay where she was.

I knelt behind her, pulled on my long plastic gloves, and did a clean-up of her rear. A careful but quick examination of her pelvic canal revealed a live calf, its head and feet both presented to the opening but wedged tight. I decided I could get the calf out without too much trouble by repositioning its head back a little to allow the legs to come out first, with the head to follow behind the knees. A quick glance toward the men revealed sadly wagging heads and grim faces. They apparently were convinced I was useless for this job, since they, three men, had not accomplished anything with their own efforts at delivering the calf. Ah, well.

I got my obstetrical chains and handles, as well as the calf puller. It's a device that strikes awe in the uninformed, as well as assisting in the delivery of calves. When the gentlemen saw the calf puller, they perked up. The calf puller was a gadget and a big one. Men love gadgets and like to think they understand them. Even if they don't understand them, they are nonetheless interested in them. At least now I had their attention.

"That machine gonna pull that calf for ye?" asked the elder Mr. Bingham, taking a long drag of his cigarette. His fingers were yellow from nicotine. He'd been smoking a long, long time.

"I'll use it if I need it," I answered. "First I have to see if I can reposition the calf so it can come out."

"You ain't gonna get it done," the old man snorted. "My boy Bobby and me been tryin' a long time. He's three times big as you. It ain't coming out, lessen you cut it out."

He dropped the nub of cigarette into the manure of the pen and ground it out with his toe. Bobby, standing next to the cow's head, shrugged in embarrassment. He was a beefy fellow, and I felt for this little cow who had endured his attempts to help her.

"We'll see," I answered.

"I've never seen a woman vet before," chimed in Mr. Garrett, leaning on the fence near Mr. Bingham. "You been doing this long?"

"Long enough," I said. I added a little more lube to my gloves.

Once back on my knees behind the cow, I inserted one arm and pushed the calf's head back a little, in order to allow room for the legs to come out first. Maneuvering the calf in very tight quarters without harming it or the cow can be quite a challenge.

This poor cow had had three men trying to extract her calf by brute force. She was tired, her vaginal canal tissue swollen, and the calf large. It was a miracle to me that the calf was still alive, but he was. When I put my finger in his mouth to test for reflexes, he grabbed on and sucked hard. That made the job a little trickier, a little more daunting. With an already dead calf, you don't have to worry about hurting it. You just have to get it out without harming the cow any more than necessary. With a live calf, you have to protect both of them. I knew I could do it, though.

In short order, I had one leg chained. I handed the end of the chain with a handle attached over to Bobby.

"Pull slow and steady," I instructed him. "Stop when I say and hold the pressure unless I say different."

Bobby was a study of concern and concentration. He easily weighed 250 pounds, all of it country-boy hard. I hoped he wouldn't pull so hard as to harm the calf.

I need not have worried. Bobby knew his strength and was so concerned about pulling too much I had to ask for a little extra from him. The first leg of the calf eased forward out of the vagina. I looped a chain on the second leg, added some more lube, and eased the second leg out. Now for the calf's head.

I slicked up my hands with the OB lube and slid them into the cow. I positioned my fingers behind the calf's ears and leaned back, pulling gently. With no more than that, I was able to usher the calf's head into the sunlight. We both rested, the calf and I, before completing the delivery. Bobby looked on, his face determined. I signaled him to begin a steady, downward pull. He complied perfectly. The shoulders of the calf were tight in the pelvis, but they popped loose from the cow after a moment or two.

Sometimes with large calves that need assistance in the birth process, the shoulders will deliver, but the hips might be a little wider, causing them to wedge in the cow's pelvis. It was always a worry for me. However, this calf was ready to get out into the world. With a little twist to position his pelvis just right, he came clear of his mama's body.

"Well, I'll be danged!" exclaimed Mr. Garrett, slapping his thigh. "She did it!"

Mr. Bingham simply sucked on a newly lit cigarette while watching silently. If he was impressed or otherwise surprised at the successful delivery, he said nothing. The calf was alive—shaking his head and flopping his long ears—and already struggling to breathe. Bobby was grinning ear-to-ear, delighted to see the wiggling calf. He took a rag from his hip pocket and began to wipe the birthing fluids and blood from the calf.

The cow was my concern now, as she was utterly exhausted and flat on her side on the ground. I checked her pelvic canal for tears and possible prolapsing tissue. Next I gave her some medication to assist in the passing of the afterbirth and some to help reduce the swelling in the pelvic canal. Sometimes after a difficult birth, the trauma to the cow will result in her becoming paralyzed in her rear legs. The paralysis might last for a day or two. Sadly, occasionally it's permanent. I went to the cow's head, took the rope that was attached to her horns, and pulled her into a sitting position.

At first she gave no indication she cared what happened to her and made no effort to remain sitting up. Bobby picked up the calf and carried it around to her head. When she saw and smelled her newborn calf, she became very animated. She began to struggle to stay up on her own. She snuffled the calf, reaching toward it with her long tongue. After a couple tries, she was able to raise herself up on shaky legs to tend to her baby. It gave me a satisfying feeling, seeing that.

Mr. Garrett, the neighbor, seemed to be surprised and happy at the results of my work.

"We messed with that cow for over two hours," he said. "I figured we were going to have to shoot her." I, for one, was glad they did not.

"Well, come on up to the house," the dour Mr. Bingham said gruffly, snuffing out still another cigarette. "Mrs. Bingham will write you a check."

I carried my equipment to the pickup and cleaned it up. While I did that, Bobby and Mr. Garrett tended to the cow and calf. They got the cow some water and feed and put some bedding down on the wet ground for the calf. It's a pretty sight, a cow licking on her wobbly calf.

Mr. Bingham waited silently for me to finish putting my equipment up, occasionally sucking on the ever-present cigarette. When I indicated I was done, he turned and led the way to the house. Silently, he held the door open for me. I walked past him into the kitchen, which was warm and smelling of fresh coffee and bread.

Mrs. Bingham was standing at the stove as we went into the tidy kitchen, and she turned to greet me with a smile. Mrs. Bingham was every bit as big and meaty as her husband was small and wizened. Jack Sprat and his wife came to mind immediately when I saw her. Mr. Bingham, another cigarette already burned down to the filter, shuffled into the kitchen. He pulled a cup out of the cabinet and poured himself some coffee, while informing his wife, in an almost bored monotone, that I was able to deliver a live bull calf to the heifer and that both cow and calf were doing well.

Mrs. Bingham was pleased with the news. She beamed a smile at me and asked me to have a seat at the kitchen table. She had a wonderful, kind face, though she obviously had some health problems that kept her in the house and moving slowly. She graciously offered me a cup of coffee, which I accepted. She produced a checkbook, shuffled over to the table, and took a chair across from me. I gave her the bill with the total on it. She studied it solemnly and carefully filled out the check.

As she handed me the check, she looked across the table at me and said, ever so quietly, "After Mr. Bingham called you and asked you to come help with the cow, he hung up the phone and said to me, 'It's a woman vet that's coming out to help us. Reckon she'll be able to do the job?'"

Mrs. Bingham leaned over the table toward me. Her eyes had gone hard, small, and mean. Lips that had smiled softly at me just a moment before were now thin and tight. I edged back from her in my chair, a little frightened.

Staring me in the eyes intently, she intoned in a dead-serious voice, "I never wanted to hit a man so much in my life."

I couldn't help it; I burst out laughing. Mrs. Bingham reared back in surprise at my response. Little Mr. Bingham, who had ducked behind his wife as she told me what he'd said, peeked at me from around her bulk, blushed, and gave a tiny smile. At first confused by my laugh, Mrs. Bingham began a slow smile that finally lit up her face, softening her features once again.

"I guess lots of people think you can't do this work because you're a woman," she said. "But who could help with birthin's better than a woman?"

❖

I remained friends with the Binghams and was their veterinarian for many years, until both of them eventually passed away from advanced age and poor health. I'll never forget that couple, their son, or the cows that I tended over the years out at the end of that long, sandy road.

Men, Women, and Cows

Animals are such agreeable friends—they ask no questions,
they pass no criticisms.
—George Eliot

There were a fair number of women in Houston County who owned cattle and ran their ranches on their own. One of my most loyal and favorite ranchers was an older woman named Pat Carroll. Pat ran a herd of good Braford cattle outside the little community of Kennard. She also produced and baled her own grass hay and bought alfalfa hay from New Mexico to supplement the winter feed for her cows. Every one of her 125 cows had a name that described some aspect of the cow.

There was one cow named Banana Head, because her long horns were shaped in smooth curves, like bananas, and bent down over her face. There was Gorgeous, who really was a beautiful cow. Number Nine had the number branded on her side, a foot tall. Sweetie liked to have her forehead rubbed. Betty Davis had large, protruding eyes.

Pat's cows were fat, healthy, and easy to work with, reflecting the temperament of their owner. Until a heart condition forced Pat to sell her cows and retire from ranching, the Serenity Ranch was one of my favorite places to go.

Other women worked their ranches with their husbands and participated fully in the operation of the ranch. Mrs. Schmidt was

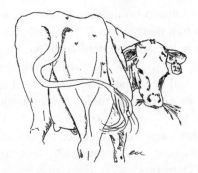

at the pens anytime I was there, taking meticulous notes on the condition of each animal. Mr. Schmidt never made a decision regarding an animal without first consulting his wife. They seemed to enjoy each other's company and worked well together.

❖

Although the sex of a cow's owner never mattered to me, the sex of the veterinarian occasionally did matter to an owner. Oddly enough, it was the women who sometimes didn't like a female veterinarian showing up to work on their cows.

Mr. and Mrs. Conrad Helms ran a registered herd of red Brangus on the far northern edge of the county. The few times I went there, it was because no other veterinarian was available. Mrs. Helms, who always referred to herself as "Mrs. Conrad Helms," never by her own given name, disapproved of women being veterinarians or holding any traditionally male jobs. She told me so each and every time I ended up attending a cow for them.

Women had no business working on a cow's "private parts" in front of men, Mrs. Conrad Helms told me. It was okay with her if I tube-wormed the horses or sewed up an injured dog. Any time I stepped behind a cow, however, she would tut-tut in disgust that I should so brazenly put my hands on the reproductive organs of a bovine. But I couldn't figure out any other way to deliver a calf or fix a prolapse.

Finally, after one difficult prolapse repair, which involved several male observers, Mrs. Helms had had enough of my blatant disregard for basic decency. As she gave me the check for the work

I'd done, she told me in no uncertain terms it was to be the last time I was to set foot on that ranch. Her husband could only shrug his shoulders in helpless agreement with her. I never did go out to that ranch again, and to make the break final, Mrs. Conrad Helms had all her cats' and dogs' medical records sent to another veterinary office, one in which only male doctors worked.

❖

Most couples who owned cattle either participated in their care on an equal basis, or it was the man who was the main caregiver to the animals. Then there were the Langleys. Mr. Langley could not be bothered with the cattle. Mrs. Langley, who insisted I call her by her baptized name, Doris, did all the cattle work while Mr. Langley stayed away from the pens, preferring to tinker in his machine shop. She favored my coming out to her ranch over any male veterinarian. She said I had more compassion and cared more than my male counterparts. She and I rarely had any problem handling her cattle.

I'll not soon forget Joe and Fanny Peters. Joe was the cattle owner in that pair, with Fanny having very little to do with the cows. I was called out one day to deliver a calf. Joe said the calf's head was out, but that was all.

"It looked dead, too," he said. "If you could come as soon as possible, I'd appreciate it. I don't want the cow to die."

I assured him I'd be there as soon as I could. When I arrived at their little ranch, Joe had the cow in his good pipe corral. There certainly was a problem. The bloated head of an obviously deceased calf showed from the cow's vagina. We sent the cow down the chute and barred her in. With soap and gloves, I examined the cow, trying to determine where the feet of the calf were. Due to the grossly swollen head, it was difficult to find the feet. Even if I'd been able to locate them, it was obvious the head would have to be removed first.

"I'll have to cut the head off the calf first, Mr. Peters," I said. "Then I'll be able to straighten the legs and pull the rest of the calf."

"Do what you gotta do," Joe replied, shaking his head at the idea of it.

About that time Fanny appeared from the direction of the house.

"Is she going to be all right?" she asked me, standing beside me, wringing her hands. I reached into the equipment box of my truck to retrieve the sharp dissecting knife with which I would remove the calf's head.

"I'm sure she will, as soon as I get this calf out of her," I replied, testing the blade of the knife for sharpness.

Fanny was a very sweet woman. She had a cat named Penny, a patient of mine. While Joe considered cats to be parasites on the human species, Fanny adored her orange-and-white cat with a passion. Any little thing that looked out of place in the cat's health had Fanny banging at the clinic door, frantic for help. Often her cause of alarm was nothing serious—a hairball, a case of ear mites picked up from the barn cats that ran wild at their ranch, or maybe fleas. I enjoyed her as a client, as her concern over the cat's well-being was based on true affection.

I walked back to the cow with my knife in hand. Joe was at the chute, and he stood to one side, holding the cow's tail out of my way. Fanny timidly moved around to get a view of what I was about to do to the calf.

"Fanny! Get back!" Joe ordered in a brusque voice. Fanny, startled, jumped a little and immediately backed up a few steps.

"Go on up to the house!" Joe snapped, trying to hold onto the cow's tail while attempting to block his wife's view of the cow's nether end. "This isn't anything a lady needs to see!"

I paused, knife raised, and looked at Joe in surprise. He turned back to me, having sent his wife scurrying back around the barn toward the house, and saw my expression.

"Oh, Doc!" he said. "I didn't mean you aren't a lady!" He turned to see his wife disappear from view. "I just meant some-one like Fanny doesn't need to see something like this!" He was blushing furiously.

I positioned the knife for my first cut behind the dead calf's head, and said nothing.

"You know what I mean, don't you?" Joe continued, trying hard to explain himself, trying hard to pull that foot out of his mouth, trying to apologize for his belief in there being a difference between his wife's status as a lady and my status as a lady veterinarian.

"Mr. Peters," I replied, deftly removing the calf's head at the first neck joint. "Don't worry about it. But maybe you ought to let Fanny see one or two things like this. Then she'll be more ready to help you out in such cases."

"Well, as long as I can find a man to help me, she doesn't need to be involved in these things," he responded, obviously without thinking. When it did occur to him what he had said, he blushed again.

"I don't mean to say you're a man," he stammered. "It's just that you're a professional. It's okay for you to see these things."

"Good thing, too," I replied. "It's hard to do this with your eyes closed."

❖

Over the years, respect for women in traditionally male roles, such as ranchers, farmers, horse trainers, and veterinarians, has increased significantly. Men in those jobs appear to have come to regard women as equals, as they should. It makes going out to do the work a lot easier, not only for the professional called upon, but for the animals that require the attention.

That is the overall good result of the persistence of women in doing the jobs they love to do.

Neither Rain Nor Hail

Cows are amongst the gentlest of breathing creatures;
none show more passionate tenderness to their young
when deprived of them; and, in short, I am not ashamed
to profess a deep love for these quiet creatures.
—Thomas De Quincey

The longer I worked in Houston County as a large-animal veterinarian, the more I came to realize how many women there were
in the ranching business. These women were not sunburned,
tobacco-chewing, hard-eyed ladies with a vendetta against men.
They were, for the most part, kind, considerate, and hard-working
individuals. They were black and they were white; they were
wives and mothers and often grandmothers; they were young and
they were elderly, as well as all ages in between. They were country women who had lived on their ranches all their born days, and
they were women who moved to the country to fulfill a dream of
owning a ranch of their own. They were educated, intelligent people who happened to be women who happened to like cattle.

I tended many cattle belonging to these women, called upon
because I was not only willing to do the job, but because I understood the woman's desire to be involved in such a job as ranching. I had empathy for the cattle, which the women appreciated,

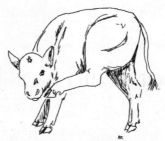

and I had empathy for the women, who were often underesti-
mated for their ability to do their jobs as ranchers.

On one early spring day, I was called out by one of these women
ranchers to help with an emergency delivery. A lot of my work with
cattle involved emergencies, and a lot of the emergencies were calf
deliveries. Calf deliveries can be quite an adrenaline rush, often
long before you get out to the ranch where the cow is. Add some
interesting weather, and the day can get very, very intense.

❖

We were having a bout of very wet weather that spring. It was still
cold enough to require heavy coats. There were occasional, torrential rains, which were sometimes preceded by hail, sometimes
followed by flooding. An office job—under a good roof with a cup
of hot coffee on a coaster near your elbow, while you sat in a
comfy chair in a climate-controlled environment—sure did seem
like a better deal on such days. While I had an office with a
coaster on my desk for my coffee cup and even an armed chair to
sit in, during calving season that chair didn't see me too often.

On this particular day the weather was reasonably warm, with
heavy clouds to the north. Away in the distance, somewhere
under the clouds, came a damp muttering of thunder. I stood at
the office window, a coffee cup in my hand, hoping the cows of the
county could control their labor urges until the storm passed by.
So far, we'd had a quiet morning, cow-wise. I could keep hoping.

Then the telephone rang. When your nerves are already tin-
gling from electricity-charged air with an accompanying feeling
of doom over such weather, a ringing phone in a large-animal

practice is particularly foreboding. I listened with one ear to what my receptionist was saying.

My heart dropped to my knees when I heard Leslie repeat to the caller, "You have a cow in trouble?"

I loved my job and actually enjoyed calf deliveries. A calf delivery is a hard, fatiguing, often nasty job, but I loved it when a calf, doomed to die in utero, would bawl lustily after being extracted in chains from his dam. I loved it when a cow in pain and also doomed if the calf wasn't delivered soon, lowed to her calf and stood up to clean it with long swipes of her raspy tongue. I loved the grin on the happy owner's face that said this year's cattle profits might not be totally down the drain after all. I really liked calf deliveries.

But I didn't like them in a cold, driving rain with lightning dancing overhead and thunder breaking on my eardrums. I didn't like those call-outs at all.

So, with trepidation in my soul, I listened more intently to the phone exchange in the other room. Leslie put the caller on hold and turned to me where I stood in the doorway.

"It's Agnes Brewer," she said. "She's got a cow down trying to calve and needs some help."

I tried, I really did, not to moan out loud. While I liked Mrs. Brewer, with her good herd of black Angus, I wasn't keen on her ranch. It was in a river bottom, and many small creek beds forked through it, making the land awkward to cross on fair days. Added to the fact that the ranch was located just about directly under where the muttering clouds were hovering, I couldn't help it—I groaned out loud.

"She says she's got a rope on the cow already," Leslie said helpfully, understanding my reluctance to jump in the truck and head out.

Leslie had been on a couple of calf deliveries with me and had been to Agnes Brewer's interesting piece of terrain. On one occasion, we'd had to abandon the truck and carry equipment across a couple of muddy creek beds and through a boot-sucking pas-

ture to reach a down cow. Leslie could see the clouds in the distance as well as I could. She was sympathetic, but also relieved
that she would not be called upon to accompany me. She was the
only employee at work that day to man the phones and the front
desk. I'd have to go this one alone. I sighed.

"Tell Mrs. Brewer that I'm on my way," I said, setting down my
coffee cup and going to the changing room to get my cow clothes
on. Leslie turned back to the phone, and I checked the sky one
more time before going to change. The clouds were still there.

Agnes Brewer's cows were well-fed individuals and used to having people around them, as Agnes was good at hand feeding cubes
to them, as well as being a gentle, easy handler. I didn't anticipate
a problem managing the cow. It was the weather that worried me.
On the drive to the ranch, twenty-five miles away, I listened to
the radio's forecast of the storm approaching and asked God to
smile, just a little, and hold off the water works until the job
ahead of us was done.

Agnes met me at the gate, a rain slicker on but not buttoned up.
She closed the gate after I had driven through, then ran around to
jump into the passenger seat. Agnes was probably sixty-five years
old, in excellent health, and every bit as agile as a woman twenty
years younger. This day she looked grim and worried.

"She's down between where the two creeks run together," she
said, jabbing her finger in a direction ahead of us. "I couldn't get
her up, but I did put a rope on her. She's about ten feet from the
edge of a drop-off. Even if she couldn't get up, I was afraid she'd
roll off the edge."

Man, I'd been there, seen that, and didn't want to again.

"You done good, Agnes," I said. "How close can we get?"

"Pretty close, actually," Agnes answered. "The pasture is fairly
dry up to a point. I'll tell you when we get there."

I drove slowly, not wishing to drop the front end of my pickup
into a shallow runoff ditch, unwilling to risk driving over the edge
of a winding creek. We drove what seemed like halfway across her
land before Agnes threw her left hand up and ordered, "Whoa."

I whoa-ed. The storm was very near, and the noontime sky was as black as ink. So far, the rain had been minute, cold spatterings of wetness with a little wind to drive it deep into the ground. In the twilight-like darkness ahead of us lay a black lump. The cow. A rope stretched between her and a pecan tree. A huge blast of thunder suddenly tore the sky open, following a lightning bolt so closely they seemed to occur simultaneously. Ahead of us, the cow appeared to leap straight up and then come down again. I jumped in my seat so high I think that without my seat belt on, I would have slammed my head into the ceiling of the cab. I think Agnes did. We looked at each other.

It was her cow, but my duty. We each had our arms wrapped tightly around our shoulders, almost as if not to touch the metal parts of the pickup. Slowly, I unfurled my arms and reached for the door handle. I swallowed and grabbed it. Better to die fast. Nothing happened. I jerked the handle, and threw the door open. The thunder rolled overhead, but no lightning strikes seemed as near as the last. I eased out of the pickup. I could see Agnes slinking forward, head ducked as if to prevent a bolt of lightning from reaching her kerchiefed head. I realized I was doing the same thing.

The ground was firm and not too muddy. I trotted as rapidly as I could in my rubber boots to the cow. Agnes had tied her so she wouldn't fall over into the ditch. She hadn't been able to make the tie-off anywhere else but on the pecan tree, however, and that tree grew within ten feet of the drop-off to the creek. Between the time Agnes had tied her off and our arrival, the cow had managed to move her labor-racked body to the edge of the drop-off. The rope had prevented her from sliding over the edge, but her rear end, the tiny front feet of an unborn calf peeking from the vulvar lips, hung over the edge of the creek.

Oh, great. What now?

Suddenly, the sky was lit so brilliantly it was as though flood lights had been turned on, blinding us, and a crack of thunder like the sound of shattering glass magnified to the tenth power split the air. It lasted at least two seconds. Fear ran a banner up my backbone and waved it. This cow had to be saved, now. While the sky still crackled from the effects of the ruptured sound barrier, and the lightning still zagged downward, I reached and grabbed the cow's tail, sat back, and pulled.

Adrenaline is a wonderful thing. Effortless it was, to swing that 900-pound body away from the creek and over to relatively dry ground. Effortless it was to roll that cow over onto her other side, so that her feet pointed away from the creek. If she tried to stand up now, she wouldn't roll into the creek. Now I could work on saving the calf. I did a quick exam of the cow. There, between the protruding hooves of the calf, a small nose was tucked. Why she couldn't deliver the calf, I didn't know.

I sprinted for the truck, expecting any moment to be struck down by a lightning bolt. I threw open the cargo space, grabbed the minimum amount of equipment necessary to do this job— chains and a set of handles—forget the gloves, soap, water. This calf was coming *before* hell and high water had a chance to reach it. I raced back to the cow, meeting Agnes halfway, as she tried to catch up with me to help. She turned in her tracks and followed me back to the cow.

I did a more thorough exam, ducking as thunder rolled. Two feet and a nose. I palpated carefully around the calf, searching for whatever was holding it fast. Ah! Two more calf feet where they shouldn't have been, under the calf's chin. I carefully traced the leg attached to one of the wayward feet. I was worried it might be a twin, trying to force its way out ahead of its sibling, but the leg proved to be a rear leg, belonging to the presenting calf. Okay, the calf was trying to jump into the world with all four feet at the same time. We could fix that.

I carefully eased one rear leg back, changed position, found the other rear leg, and eased it back into the cow's uterus. Suddenly the cow grunted, strained, and the calf literally flew out of her in a heap on the ground beside me.

Was it alive? Yes! Stunned for a moment, it gave a bawl and shook its head. The cow came up to the sternal position and turned her head so she could see the calf. She sang out a long, relieved moo.

Lightning tore across the land, and thunder broke open the sky. Rain fell, so hard it felt like glass shards. Agnes and I both shrieked in terror and distress. I grabbed the calf by its back legs and ran, dragging it toward the truck. The cow behind us gave a bellow at my theft of her calf and lunged to her feet. The rope held her firmly to the tree. At the truck I attempted to pick up the slippery sixty pounds of newborn calf to get it on the tailgate. I looked back to see where Agnes was. She was at the pecan tree, frantically sawing with a pocketknife at the rope that still held her cow, now up and fighting her restraint.

The rope popped in two, the cow staggered back a foot or two, and then turned, bawled into the pouring rain, and started trotting toward the truck and her calf. Agnes ran, too, slowing slightly to scoop up the chains and handles I had left lying near the cow. She galloped up beside me, tossing the equipment into the bed. Together we hefted the wiggling calf up onto the truck, rain pelting us, the cow trying to lick the calf. Agnes nimbly leapt up and landed bottom first on the tailgate next to the calf, feet over the edge. She grabbed the calf firmly under one arm, and latched the fingers of her other hand tightly on the side rail of the truck.

"Drive! Drive!" she screamed over the storm. I raced to the cab, leapt in, cranked the engine, and floored it. In the rearview mirror I saw Agnes lurch but hold steady. Behind us, the cow was coming, while the truck's spinning tires flung mud all over her face and chest. She never slowed down, but bellowed indignantly and followed her truck-riding calf at a trot.

I don't know how we got out of that muddy pasture, except maybe by the grace of God and a team of his hardest working angels, but we did. We drove up to the gate Agnes had latched shut earlier, and I threw the truck into park, jumped out, ran to the gate, swung it wide, ran back to the truck, and jumped in again. The cow had barely caught up with us as I gassed the engine again, once again spewing her with mud off the rear tires.

She didn't seem to care; as long as her calf was moving away from her, she was going to try to catch up.

We must have taken the turn into the barnyard on two wheels. I don't know how Agnes managed to stay on board, while clinging to a slimy newborn calf, but she did. She jumped off the tailgate. The cow skidded to a halt beside her calf, singing her cow song, snuffling her offspring, spraying muddy water with her breath from the pouring rain that ran off her nose. Agnes ran and opened the barn door, and I dragged the lively calf into the barn. A horse stall would provide shelter for the calf. The cow came as far as the door, stuck her head in, lowed at the calf, and then followed it into the stall. The cow was so focused on her calf she paid me no mind as I scurried past her and out of the stall. Agnes swung the stall door closed as I scooted out.

For a few minutes we two women stood leaning against the wall, heaving in great lungfuls of air, water cascading from our heads and clothing. Agnes never had taken the time to snap her rain slicker closed, and she was almost as wet as I was. I was totally drenched, head to toe, the water having run into my boots as well as soaking me to the skin. We looked at each other, assessed each other, and both of us burst out laughing at the same time. What an adventure!

The cow was licking her calf vigorously, and the calf was protesting in squeaky calf bawls. He struggled to get to his feet. Both Agnes and I were delighted to have rescued both the cow and the calf, but the cold rainwater soaking us was taking its toll. I was starting to shake like a leaf. My fingers were turning blue, and I figured if I looked half as miserable as I felt, I was looking pretty bad. Agnes had drawn her slicker tight around herself and was vibrating from the chill.

"We have to get the rope off the cow," I said through chattering teeth.

Agnes waved her hand in dismissal.

"I'll get it off her later," she said, "when I come back to give her some hay and water. Let's you and me get to the house and have some hot tea."

I eagerly accepted. I knew she'd give me a towel and a dry shirt. We opened the barn door and gazed out into the driving rain toward her house, which looked a hundred miles away. About that time, the rain slacked up considerably. We dashed for the house.

Agnes set the kettle on the stove while I toweled my hair. She had cranked the house's heat system up to high. She was still quite excited about the outcome of the call-out and threw in an apology every now and again, for the weather, for having to call me, for my current soaked state … as if any of it was her fault. I was so happy to be inside, out of the rain, I almost didn't mind that I was still drenched and cold. The anticipation of a cup of hot tea was already warming me up from the inside.

Just as the kettle began to whistle, Agnes' phone rang. She set the two cups she had gotten down from the cabinet on the table and answered the phone.

"Hello?" she said, wiping her hands on a cloth. "Dr. Cooper-Chase? Yes, she's still here. Hold on a minute." Agnes turned toward me. She passed the phone to me.

"It's your office," she said, apparently not picking up on my look of dismay. I took the phone tentatively from her.

It was Leslie. She was very apologetic, but another client had an animal in trouble.

"Who and what?" I asked.

"Mrs. Wyatt," she answered. "She's got a cow trying to calve."

I blanched. I looked out the window of Agnes' kitchen. The storm was passing by, but it was headed down the road and probably getting ready to set up camp over Mrs. Margaret Wyatt's ranch, south of where I sat in Agnes Brewer's kitchen.

"Tell her," I said slowly, not really wanting to say it, "tell her I'll be there as soon as possible."

I hung up the phone. Agnes looked extremely sympathetic as she held the steaming cup of tea out to me.

"Take it with you," she said. "I'll get the cup next time I come to town."

I nodded numbly, gratefully took the life-giving cup, and walked to the door. The rain had stopped coming down over the

Agnes Brewer homestead. South of us, in the direction I must now travel, the heavy black clouds boiled and rolled, lightning flashing from their depths. I took a deep breath, stumbled outside to the truck, got in, cranked the motor, slid the heater knob to full blast, put the truck in reverse, waved at Agnes, and pulled out of her yard.

❖

The truck heater did its best, but the rain had been cold and drenching, and I shivered uncontrollably in my wet clothes as I drove. It was thirty miles to Margaret Wyatt's place. She was another of my good female ranchers. Where were the men, I wondered crossly? Why were women the only ones out checking their cows in the rain? Were the men safe inside, huddled down with hot drinks, chuckling over the foolhardiness of women ranchers? I fumed a little over my perceived injustice of it and picked up speed a little, racing the clouds to the Wyatt place.

The scenario at Margaret's was pretty much like it had been at Agnes'—the black clouds scudding low and the sky at just past midday looking very much like late-evening instead. But, Oh, Joy! Margaret's twelve-year-old son, Robbie, was at the gate, holding it open for me, so I didn't have to exit the truck to open it. Margaret's ranch was on higher ground, and I expected it to be a little drier. I drove through the gate and stopped, waiting for Robbie to close the gate and climb into the passenger seat. Robbie was a good boy, helpful to his mother, and a bona fide talker. He was already chatting excitedly as he hopped into the truck.

"Mom's with the cow!" he crowed. "It's old Vanessa. She won't get up. Mom thinks the calf is backwards!" He stopped to draw breath.

"Where is she?" I asked quickly.

"The Bottom!" he answered. "She laid down in the dry creek bed a couple of hours ago, but it started flooding, and Mom couldn't get her to stand up and get out of the water!"

Oh, my. I put the pedal to the metal, and the truck lurched forward, bouncing over the rough ground. Robbie was having a good time, hanging on to his seat as the truck rose and fell on the irregular ground. He directed me over the field and through a couple of gates, to a pasture that dipped down toward a normally dry creek bed, a creek bed that didn't see water unless the rains had come hard farther upstream. I had been "upstream" and had seen the rains come. Overhead, the clouds circled, as if looking for just the right place to drop their payload. On the ground, water was coursing across the pasture, heading for the cow and the woman in the creek.

Vanessa was an old cow, just like Robbie said. I had been thinking she wasn't going to make it another year for the past three years now. She had been Margaret's high school show calf, and Margaret had a deep, abiding love and respect for the old Brangus-cross cow. Most of Vanessa's deep-red hair had faded to an orangey hue as advancing age gradually replaced it with white hair. I figured she had to be at least nineteen years old. She was far too old to be calving in a wet pasture bottom.

As if reading my thoughts, Robbie spoke up.

"Mom had her in the pen for two weeks now," he informed me. "She didn't act like she was ever going to have that calf, so Mom let her out to graze down here for a little while. When she didn't come back this morning, we had to find her. Mom found her lying down in the creek bed. You couldn't even see her at first. We got her to go this far, before she lay down again and wouldn't get up. Mom came back to the house to call you."

I could see the cow and her owner ahead of us. We bounced to a halt next to the cow. Upon seeing a strange vehicle in her vicinity, the cow sat up onto her chest and swung her old, long face toward us. She was a terribly sad-looking cow. Margaret jogged over to the truck.

"She broke water about two hours ago," she said, as I climbed stiffly out of my truck. Apparently neither she nor Robbie noticed I was still soaking wet, my clothes plastered to me. I was shivering slightly. My hair was still dripping water, in spite of the toweling I'd given it in Agnes' kitchen. Their concern was for their own cow.

"I couldn't get her to stand up at first," Margaret continued. "She had a real hard time getting this far, but she fell here, and that's it." She pointed to the north. "Storm's coming, too," she added about the obvious.

The clouds looked like they were coming in for a landing. Water from rains farther north were cascading down the creek bed, and the stream was divided by the bulk of the cow, who lay still on her chest, her thoughts turned inward to the wrongly positioned calf.

"Let's try to get her out of here," I said, and together we urged the cow to rise with slaps and whoops. She gave a half-hearted lunge and settled back down on the ground. I ran to my truck for my equipment, Robbie pacing me, coming to help carry things I might need.

At that moment, as I handed some small things to Robbie, a sharp "ping!" sounded, then another, and another. Hail was pelting us and pinging off the metal of the truck.

"Robbie! Get in the truck!" I shouted. "Margaret! Come get in the truck! It's hailing!"

Robbie was already in the cab, and the hailstones, not bigger than marbles, began to bang down in earnest. I shielded my head and ducked into the cab with Robbie.

Unbelievably, Margaret was not only staying out in the storm, she was standing up, hunched over, holding her rain coat over Vanessa's head, shielding her from the stinging pellets of ice. The cow never moved, nor did the woman, as the ice shower beat over them. In just a few minutes, it passed. We got out of the pickup. The ground was white with ice balls, small and slippery. Robbie trotted toward his mother.

From the north came a roar. We looked in that direction. Margaret lowered her coat and straightened up, turning with her son and me to see what was coming.

Water. A wall of water about three feet high was coursing down the dry creek bed. It carried sticks and small logs and rafts of woodland trash made up of leaves and pine needles. It roared down the pasture in a brown torrent. Robbie did not need instructions to get in the pickup. He turned and ran and almost dived through the door of the truck into the seat.

"Margaret!" I screamed. "GET UP HERE!"

The water was coming fast. I ran down as close to the cow and the woman as I could.

"MARGARET!" I called again.

She waved me back and slogged through the water to the head of her beloved cow. She took the cow's chin, raised it high, and set it on her own shoulder. She wrapped her arms firmly around the cow's neck and clasped her hands together tightly. And she stood there and waited for the brown flood to hit them.

I had no idea what to do. I could only wonder, what was she thinking? Could she really believe she could save this old, crippled cow? Did she really want to die like that in front of her young son?

The water hit the rear of the cow, splashed and parted around her, washed over her back, and slammed into Margaret. The cow disappeared. The woman's head stayed up a moment, and then the pull of the water flipped her backwards and down she went, still holding that cow's neck.

I put my hands over my mouth, afraid to scream, afraid to look back and see Robbie's frightened face, afraid of what I would see as the water slowed and receded and banked away from the higher rolls of the pasture.

Almost as quickly as it hit, the wall of water disappeared, churning down the creek, taking its trash along with it. And surfacing maybe fifteen feet farther downstream was a reddish cow with a woman clinging desperately to her neck.

I ran as fast as I could toward them. Behind me I heard the truck door open and slam closed, and the running of a young boy's feet. He never uttered a word.

We got to the cow. Margaret was choking and gasping and spitting out dirty brown water. A fine trickle of blood flowed from a minor gash on her forehead. She slowly relinquished her grip on her cow.

And Vanessa mooed, long and low, and shook her long ears to rid them of the water in them. She was on slightly higher ground, and the water was returning to its former level of twelve inches.

Margaret grabbed her son and hugged him fiercely, and he clung to her wet clothes desperately.

"Did you see what your mama did?" Margaret asked her son, holding his face between her hands and looking him right in the eye. "Did you see that?"

He nodded numbly.

"Good," she said. "And I don't EVER want you to do anything even remotely as stupid as that as long as you live." She patted his shoulder fiercely, fondly, and then turned to me.

"Can we save the calf?" she asked.

I was speechless from what I'd just seen. I looked at the cow, who regarded me gravely. She grunted and strained. Nothing showed.

"Come on, Robbie," I said. "We have to deliver this calf before the rain starts falling in earnest." We ran for the truck, got the equipment and supplies we needed, and ran back to the cow.

Fortunately enough, although it was a breech presentation, the calf was small with lots of room to move around in the cow. As lightning flashed and thunder threatened, I lay behind the cow on the cold, wet ground, working to deliver the calf. Thunder boomed in response to a close-by lightning bolt, and I asked Margaret and Robbie to get to the safety of the truck. I'd have the calf in a minute. Robbie turned and ran for the truck like a scared rabbit, but Margaret lingered.

Lightning flared again, and Margaret fell hard, flattened out on the ground beside me. At first, due to the extreme stress I was under, I thought Margaret had been struck by the lightning. When she slid her arms off her head and raised her widened, scared eyes to me, I knew that it wasn't so. She took a chain handle and indicated she was willing to stay and help deliver the calf. I wasn't going to refuse her help. I got one of the calf's legs in position and then the other, and in a minute a little heifer calf slid into the world.

No sooner did we have the chains off the calf than the sky opened and dropped its heavy burden of rain. It felt more like a waterfall than a rainstorm. We dragged and slid the calf toward the truck, and heaved it into the bed. Behind us, Vanessa bawled for her calf and struggled gallantly to her feet. She had a little wobble in her rear legs, but without the calf pressing down on the nerves in her pelvis, she was able to stand and walk. The muddy ground slowed her just a little as she hurried after her calf.

"Robbie!" I hollered. "Can you drive this truck?"

"Yes, ma'am!" he answered strongly.

"Can he?" I asked Margaret.

She nodded. "He can drive anything," she said.

"Robbie!" I hollered. "Get us out of here!"

While he slid excitedly over to the driver's side, I got my equipment, pitched it into the bed of the truck, and hopped up on the tailgate next to Margaret, who sat clutching the calf, bent over, shielding it from the worst of the rain. The cow would follow the truck.

Robbie did a good job of getting the truck back to the front gate without getting us stuck or causing either of us, or the calf, to bounce off the tailgate. By the time we got to the road, the rain had abated somewhat. In short order the cow and calf were safely stashed under a lean-to near the house.

I don't know if Margaret was aware of me at all. She was deeply concerned with her cow and calf, though obviously relieved and happy to have both of them safe. She sent Robbie after towels to dry the calf and hay and water for the cow. I waited a little, delighted to see the newborn calf snorting and shaking the water off its head. I was soaking wet and freezing, though, and backed away to my pickup, climbed aboard, and drove out of the farmyard, heading for home. What a day.

Margaret stopped by the clinic the following morning, embarrassed for not having offered me a hot drink and a towel and forgetting to pay her bill. I wasn't worried about it. Folks with that much concern for a simple beast such as a cow will almost always come around and take care of their affairs later.

❖

I could always work for people like Margaret Wyatt and Agnes Brewer and folks like the Drummonds, the Duvalls, Ronald Bryan, and even Mr. Martin. There were many other good men and women, too, whom I haven't mentioned in these stories. Their care and concern for the animals under their husbandry are what I remember most about the call-outs to assist in veterinary medical crises and routine procedures. They're the kind of people I miss and who make me miss my large-animal practice.

The cold and the damp, the heat with its headaches and sweat, the sore muscles and enormous fatigue, the bad roads and long hours take a back seat in my memory banks when I recall the creatures and the many good people who asked for my help.

About the Author

Animals have always played a significant part in the life of Rosalie Cooper-Chase. Growing up in a family with ten children, Rosalie spent weekends while in high school working at a horse farm, where she also started her association with cattle by milking dairy cows.

Later, as a vet assistant, Rosalie took night classes and saved enough money to become a full-time college student. When funds ran low, she returned to her vet assistant work and began saving again. In 1982, she was admitted into the veterinary medicine curriculum at Texas A&M, graduating in 1986.

Rosalie began her career in San Antonio and then purchased the South Pine Animal Hospital in Crockett, Texas, where she still practices today.

Although injuries forced her to give up her large-animal veterinary work, Rosalie still rides her horses on the small ranch where she and her husband Jack live, along with numerous cats and two dogs. She keeps a few head of cattle at a friend's place nearby.